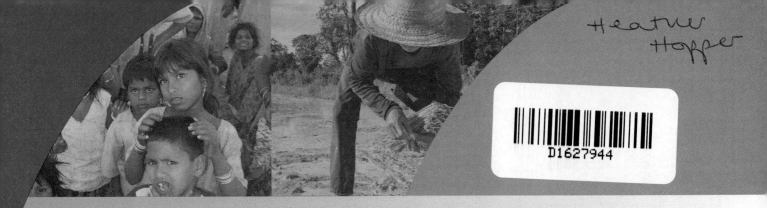

Essentials of Health, Culture, and Diversity

Understanding People, Reducing Disparities

Mark Edberg, PhD

Associate Professor
Department of Prevention and Community Health
School of Public Health and Health Services
Joint Appointment, Department of Anthropology
The George Washington University
Washington, DC

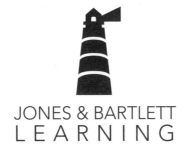

JONES & BARTLETT
LEARNING

World Headquarters
Jones & Bartlett Learning
5 Wall Street
Burlington, MA 01803
978-443-5000
info@jblearning.com
www.jblearning.com

Jones & Bartlett Learning books and products are available through most bookstores and online booksellers. To contact Jones & Bartlett Learning directly, call 800-832-0034, fax 978-443-8000, or visit our website, www.jblearning.com.

Substantial discounts on bulk quantities of Jones & Bartlett Learning publications are available to corporations, professional associations, and other qualified organizations. For details and specific discount information, contact the special sales department at Jones & Bartlett Learning via the above contact information or send an email to specialsales@jblearning.com.

This publication is designed to provide accurate and authoritative information in regard to the Subject Matter covered. It is sold with the understanding that the publisher is not engaged in rendering legal, accounting, or other professional service. If legal advice or other expert assistance is required, the service of a competent professional person should be sought.

Some images in this book feature models. These models do not necessarily endorse, represent, or participate in the activities represented in the images.

Production Credits
Publisher: Michael Brown
Editorial Assistant: Teresa Reilly
Editorial Assistant: Chloe Falivene
Production Assistant: Rebekah Linga
Senior Marketing Manager: Sophie Fleck Teague
Manufacturing and Inventory Control Supervisor: Amy Bacus
Composition: Publishers' Design and Production Services, Inc.
Cover Design: Kristin E. Parker

Photo Researcher: Sarah Cebulski
Cover and Chapter Opener Images: Children begging on the street: © Nikhil Gangavane/Dreamstime.com; Indian grandmother with child: © Indianeye/Dreamstime.com; Workers in rice field: © Mcpics/Dreamstime.com; People bathing in ocean: © Ashish Maurya/Dreamstime.com
Printing and Binding: Malloy, Inc.
Cover Printing: Malloy, Inc.

Library of Congress Cataloging-in-Publication Data
Edberg, Mark Cameron, 1955-
  Essentials of health, culture, and diversity : understanding people, reducing disparities / Mark Edberg. -- 1st ed.
    p. cm.
  Includes bibliographical references and index.
  ISBN 978-0-7637-8045-6 (pbk.) -- ISBN 0-7637-8045-6 (ibid.) 1. Social medicine. 2. Health services accessibility. I. Title.
  RA418.E327 2013
  362.1--dc23
                                                                                                    2011042560

6048

Printed in the United States of America
16 15 14 13 12   10 9 8 7 6 5 4 3 21

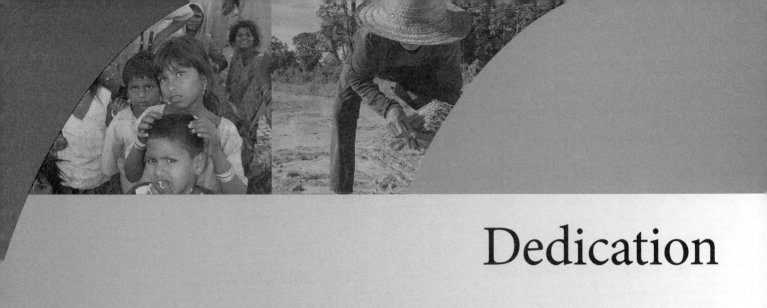

Dedication

This book is dedicated to my family for their support and tolerance, to all those at The George Washington University and at Jones & Bartlett Learning who are behind the *Essential Public Health* series and related volumes, and, importantly, to all those already working or planning to work on the front lines to help improve the lives and health of so many people in the United States and around the world. Your work is a testament to humanity at its best.

Mark Edberg, PhD
The George Washington University

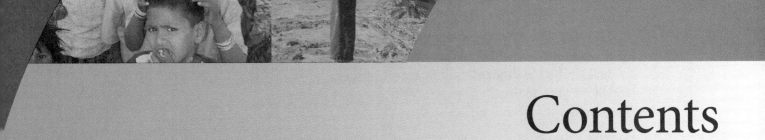

Contents

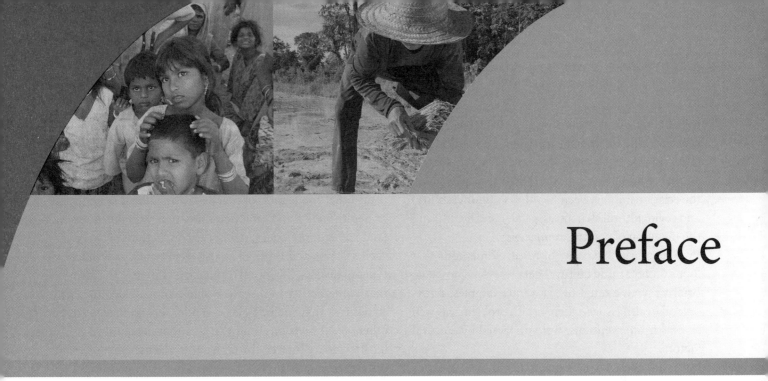

Preface

HEALTH, CULTURE, AND DIVERSITY: UNDERSTANDING PEOPLE, REDUCING DISPARITIES

The term *culture* has increasingly been used in the discourse of public health, for example, with respect to issues of health disparities in the United States, and the development and implementation of culturally competent or culturally appropriate programs to name a few. What exactly *is* culture, however? The term is easily applied to all kinds of phenomena, without a critical look at the nature of and role of culture as an aspect of human behavior. This book will examine what is meant by culture, the ways in which culture intersects with health issues, how public health efforts—especially efforts to reduce health disparities in both domestic and global settings—can benefit by understanding and working with cultural processes, and a selection of conceptual tools and research methods that are useful in identifying relationships between culture and health. The book also includes practical guidelines for incorporating cultural understanding in public health settings, and examples of programs where that has occurred.

A focus on culture and its relationship to health fills an important gap for undergraduate programs in public health and will provide an important part of the foundation necessary for understanding the field. There are few current (undergraduate) texts that (1) provide a broad introduction to the concept of culture; (2) reframe the general concept of culture as a set of tools or lenses through which health knowledge, health behavior, social institutions and practices related to health, and the nature of health risk can be understood; and (3) apply these cultural tools to a range of public health issues, both domestic and global, including practical, program-related applications. This book does all three.

It is almost axiomatic that current and future students of public health need to have a better understanding of the role of culture. Not only is the U.S. population becoming more diverse, but the separation between domestic and global public health applications has become less meaningful. Diversity, including cultural diversity, is the norm. Thus, in this evolving environment, students and others planning to work in public health should have more than a cursory understanding of the important cultural dimension of the human societies and groups with whom they will be partners.

Health, Culture, and Diversity is designed to:

1. Introduce the concept of culture as one framework for understanding human behavior. Based on that concept, to introduce the general relationship between culture and health.

2. Provide an overview of specific domains where culture and health intersect, using a range of conceptual tools. These include: varying definitions of health/

well-being; understandings of health risk; illness causation and treatment theories (ethnomedical and ethnopsychiatric systems); healing/curing traditions; culture, illness, and morality (the roots of stigma); the relationship between health risk (vulnerability) and sociocultural structures; gender and health; and the meaning of *cultural competency*.

3. Provide a brief overview of research methods that focus on obtaining cultural data.

4. Briefly review a range of cases and examples, across several health issues, where health problems, as well as health interventions, were impacted by cultural factors.

5. Focus on three current public health issues where culture and health intersect: HIV/AIDS, obesity, and youth violence.

6. Generally explore some of the ways in which an awareness of the culture–health relationship can inform public health work, both domestically and internationally.

7. Expand the reader's understanding of *cultural competency* so that it encompasses a broad spectrum of relationships between culture, health, and well-being.

The first section introduces the concept of culture, not only through the analysis of definitions and specific features, but by presenting the idea in a broad sense—as a key aspect of what makes us human. Culture will be connected to the way all humans interpret and make sense of life, to the way we are socially organized and carry out our daily tasks, and as a key source of motivation for behavior—including health-related behavior. In the second section, the connections between culture and health will be clarified through the use of several conceptual tools and approaches—the idea of systems of health belief and practice known as *ethnomedical* (and *ethnopsychiatric*) *systems*; the connections between such systems and types of health treatments, as well as types of healers; the moral dimension of illness; the idea that vulnerability to disease is shaped by sociocultural structures that include class, gender, economics, and other social divisions; and the idea that perceptions of health risk are filtered through cultural lenses that offer different answers to the question *what is a health risk?* In the third section, the book takes an in-depth look at several examples of health issues that are significantly impacted by cultural factors: HIV/AIDS, obesity (and its consequences), and youth violence. It then provides an overview of practical strategies and approaches for identifying cultural factors that affect health conditions, and working with these factors to develop and implement public health interventions that make sense in context and are more likely to be effective. Finally, this section reviews the concept and practice of cultural competence and its role in reducing health disparities. Throughout, the book includes real-life examples and profiles, as well as suggested exercises and activities to help in understanding concepts and their application.

Mark Edberg, PhD

Prologue

Eliminating health disparities has been a national goal since *Healthy People* announced its importance at the dawn of the 21st century. Yet as each year passes, the issue of health disparities takes on new importance and gains new attention as public health recognizes the central role played by social and cultural determinants of health.

Understanding health disparities requires that we go back to basics and ask fundamental questions about what we mean by health, what we mean by culture, and what we mean by diversity. That is exactly what Mark Edberg does in his new book, *Essentials of Health, Culture, and Diversity: Understanding People, Reducing Disparities*. This new book for the *Essential Public Health* series is written in the same engaging and thought-provoking style that has made Dr. Edberg's other book, *Essentials of Health Behavior*, a widely acclaimed text that is well on its way to becoming a classic.

Dr. Edberg's education as an anthropologist provides the grounding for him to venture forth into territory that needs to be addressed by public health or healthcare education. Cultural competence takes on new and expanded meaning as he explores the ways that culture affects the health risks we take, the ways we respond to illness, and the strategies we use to address public health issues.

Essentials of Health, Culture, and Diversity: Understanding People, Reducing Disparities is structured as a textbook, ideal for a one-semester or one-quarter course. Both undergraduate and graduate students will benefit. Dr. Edberg applies his extensive experience teaching in this new text, using a wide range of classroom-tested teaching methods. The book stands on its own with all the theoretical and practical background needed to address the issues and teach a course.

Dr. Edberg is able to bring behavioral theories to life by providing relevant examples and extended case studies. To illustrate his approach, Dr. Edberg focuses on HIV/AIDS, obesity, and youth violence to provide in-depth understanding of these key public health issues.

As editor of the *Essential Public Health* series, I am delighted that Mark Edberg has again applied his talents to a subject central to the way we look at public health and health care. I'm confident that *Essentials of Health, Culture, and Diversity: Understanding People, Reducing Disparities* will give you new perspectives and new understandings that you can use every day.

Richard Riegelman, MD, PhD
Editor, *Essential Public Health* series

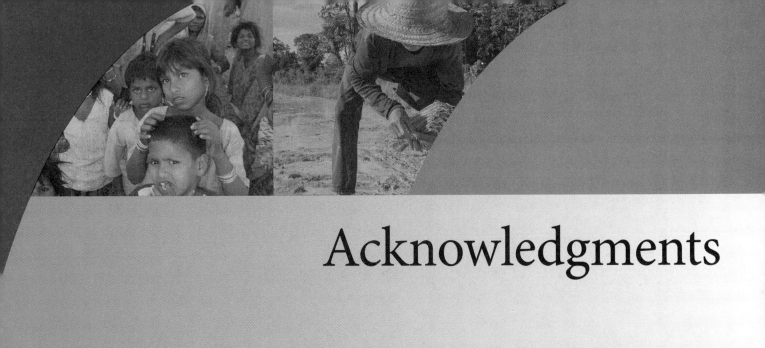

Acknowledgments

I am deeply grateful to a number of individuals and others who provided invaluable support and assistance in preparing this book:

1. Dr. Richard Riegelman, for his leadership in compiling the series and for shepherding everyone through the process.
2. Allison Harvey, for MPH, and Neela Satyanarayana, MPH, their herculean efforts in finding all kinds of material (from articles to data and photos), research support, and developing charts and graphics—often from loose descriptions and drawings.
3. Laurie Krieger, PhD, for assistance with an interview that appears in Chapter 11.
4. The Department of Prevention and Community Health, School of Public Health and Health Services at The George Washington University, for overall support and expertise, and the Department of Anthropology, for maintaining the connection between the material in this book and its roots in anthropological inquiry.

And of course, many thanks to my wife, Haykham, and children, Eleazar and Jordana, for tolerating the constant and time-consuming work that is involved in putting together a book, and for humoring the occasional monologue that seems to accompany the process.

Mark Edberg, PhD

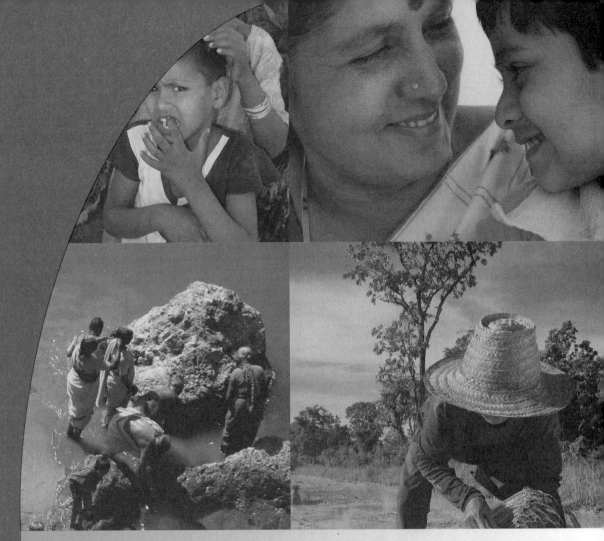

SECTION ONE

Culture and the Human Condition—An Introduction

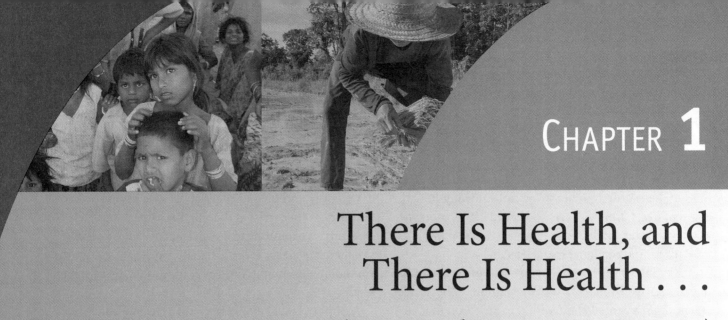

CHAPTER 1

There Is Health, and There Is Health . . .

(Laura Smith Encounters a Situation)

Let's engage in an imaginative exercise. Think of a person—let's call her Laura Smith. Of course you don't know much about her at this point, but let's just say she comes from a family of medical practitioners in Phoenix, Arizona, and though she is not a medical professional (in fact, she is a graduate student in New York), she is relatively well versed in biomedical knowledge.

But today, she is not in Arizona, or New York. She is in another country. And today, she doesn't feel well. In fact, she feels *sick*. She is throwing up, and seems to have a fever, and in addition, her side hurts and her feet feel swollen. So as she suffers in her hotel room, she searches in her mind for an explanation, a label. She wants to know what to call her sickness. *OK, what exactly is wrong here . . . ?* In her mind, she goes through a checklist of her symptoms and tries to connect them to a cause. *Did I eat something bad? Hmmm, maybe the shrimp I had last night. After all, seafood that isn't fresh can cause problems. Or was I around someone who had a virus, like the flu, that I caught? Were they coughing? Hmmm, did I get an insect bite? Was it a virus or bacteria from an insect bite? Ahh, maybe the water . . . but no, I'm pretty sure I drank only bottled water.*

Not arriving at a satisfactory connection, she goes downstairs to the hotel desk. This particular hotel is not a major chain, or even a big hotel, but a small, local hotel. Using sign language and whatever else she can to communicate, she manages to get across to the desk clerk that she needs a doctor of some kind. He smiles reassuringly, and points down the road, giving her an address. So she walks, still feeling weak, to the corner of the block and to the address she was given. It looks like a small store. She frowns and looks around, quizzically, and proceeds into the store, showing the address to an old woman behind the counter who points up a set of stairs. Shaking her head and muttering, Laura makes her way up the stairs to an office that has a strange icon on the door and in English, as well as other languages, the words "Healing Arts." Somewhat desperate at this point, she opens the door and enters. *OK, at least it looks like a waiting room. There is a counter, and someone behind it.* The woman behind the counter motions her to sit down.

About 10 minutes later, the door next to the counter opens and a short man with his gray hair in a long ponytail pokes his head out. He bows his head and motions for her to come in.

Laura asks, right away, "Do you speak any English?" He nods, and she breathes a sigh of relief.

"Tell me," he says in a low, but soothing voice, accented but clear enough for her to understand, "what is the problem?" She describes her symptoms and the healer nods his head. Then he asks her a few questions. "Tell me, why are you traveling here?" *An odd question, but I'll answer.* "Well, I have an internship in Indonesia, you know, for graduate school, and I thought I'd take a few stops on the way and see some things I have wanted to see. I even have a list."

The healer nods his head. "Ah, so you are in a hurry?" Laura furrows her brow, not knowing how to answer. "Yes, I think you are. You have a list. Now, let me ask you . . . this graduate internship, what is it for?"

"It's for international management."

"Ah, international management. Yes, you would like to manage. Well then, wait one minute." The healer reaches into a carved chest with the same icon that appeared on the door. He pulls out a long wooden dowel with a disk at one end covered in symbols and some kind of language. "Please, lay back." As he brings out the dowel, he lights two or three candles that burn with a strong aromatic fragrance. He takes the dowel with its disk-symbol, and proceeds to wave it slowly back and forth up her body, from her feet to her head. He puts the dowel away and holds her wrist, closing his eyes, then taking her other wrist and doing the same.

Laura is beginning to feel alarmed. *What is he doing? What kind of doctor is this?* "Excuse me, what exactly are you doing? I thought you were, like, a doctor of some kind!"

"Shhhh. I am, I am. Just be still." He then holds each of her ankles, this time humming what seems to be a quiet chant. "Please sit up now." Puzzled, Laura follows his direction. "Just a few more questions. Can you tell me, when

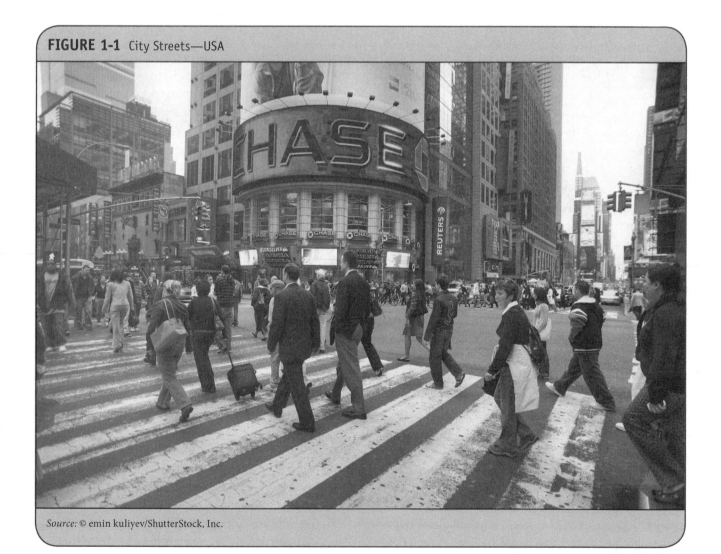

FIGURE 1-1 City Streets—USA

Source: © emin kuliyev/ShutterStock, Inc.

you are in your country, what is your typical day? By this, when you get up, what you do, things of this type?"

By this point, Laura is tired and simply goes along with the process. "Let's see, I get up at 7 a.m., eat a quick breakfast . . ."

"What do you eat?" he interjects.

She finds herself strangely willing to talk. "I don't know, maybe a bagel and cream cheese, maybe a bowl of cereal. Then I rush out the door to catch a bus to the subway. Sometimes I'm late so I run. Then I get to work and go and get a cup of coffee before I go to my office—I work part time at an import-export company while I'm in graduate school. Then I try to catch up with the pile of forms and papers on my desk because at 2 in the afternoon I have to go to class . . ."

"Do you eat in the middle of the day, lunch?"

"Oh yeah, lunch. I run back downstairs and grab a sandwich, oh any kind, ham and cheese, whatever, and a soda, maybe a candy bar for energy. Anyway, then I go to class at 2 until 5, and usually come back to work for an hour or two to finish up, and then, let's see, I get on the subway to go back home, or some days I stay at the library 'til about 10 p.m., then go home. Sometimes I wish I had a car. At home I . . ."

"Do you eat in the evening?"

"Oh, yeah, dinner. Geez, I don't even know. Um, I make up something quickly when I get home or get some soup and salad at the supermarket, or get some take-out Chinese food."

"Do you talk to anybody? Do you see family?"

"What? Oh, once in a while I catch a movie with a couple of friends. I text them, they text me. I live in New York, and my family lives in Arizona . . . that, if you don't know, is almost on the other side of the country, and in the south."

"I see. Please sit a minute." The old man walks back through the door and returns with three plastic bags, each containing what looks like herbs, or in one case, leaves. He opens his cabinet and pulls out a small version of his wooden dowel with the circular disk, and gives it to Laura. "Here is what I would like you to do. Please go back to where you are staying, and open the window, but close the curtains. Put a blanket on the floor, and sit on it comfortably. Place the healing stick

I just gave to you in front of you, but not too close, so that it stands up with the disk at the top. Close your eyes and focus on the picture of the healing stick. Do this for a little while. Then get up, and go outside for a walk. Do not eat. When you come back, make yourself a tea with these (he hands her the bag with leaves in it), but let it cool before you drink it. You may then eat, but eat nothing hot. Only cold food. Before you go to bed, mix this powder (he hands her a bag with a reddish-brown powder) with a little cold water and rub this on your stomach and your head, like this (he demonstrates a self-massage technique). In the morning, make yourself the tea again, and drink when cool. Sit on the blanket, close your eyes, and think of the healing stick again. If you plan to leave to go to a new place tomorrow, wait one day before leaving. If you still do not feel good, place a small amount of this (hands her the third bag with a green powder in it) in a cup of cold water and drink it. Sit on the blanket again, but this powder may make you fall asleep. When you wake up, make the cold tea again." The old man smiles.

Laura looks at him as if he were a character in a movie. "What?"

He nods his head, expecting her reaction. "Please, do as I ask. Your body is like the weather. It has seasons, some hot, some cold, but they always are a balance to each other. We have names for these seasons of the body, but I don't think you want to know them. You have created many hot seasons in your body, and this has caused the different parts of your body to act in the wrong way to each other, like a family arguing. Or, you could say like a storm that is created when a hot wind blows into a cold one. What I have told you will restore your balance, for now. After that it is up to you . . . You want to manage, and you must first know how to manage yourself."

Laura is slightly annoyed by the last comment. But she takes the materials and when she is about to leave, she asks, "Oh, I'm sorry, what do I owe you?" She fumbles for her wallet.

The old man smiles. "Ah yes. Not money. Ask the old woman downstairs to prepare me a good meal, and she will tell you how much she wants for that." Laura mutters under her breath. As she steps out of the office, she almost bumps in to what looks like a family sitting in the chairs, clearly waiting to be seen.

There are two young boys, in threadbare robes, and a woman with her hair up in a tight bun who is on her knees in the corner of the waiting room, placing a small bouquet of flowers into a cup of water next to a kind of altar, underneath a carved and painted figurine that is completely unfamiliar to Laura.

The woman is wearing a robe and a faded shawl. She looks up, appearing to control her surprise at seeing someone like Laura in that office. *Locals? Native Indians from around here?* Laura wonders to herself. *They must believe in this stuff.* For a moment, she has a strong urge to throw the bags of herbs and other materials on the floor and stomp out in disgust. But she doesn't want to make a scene and smiles weakly at the woman, who is still looking at her.

After walking out of the store downstairs and paying the old woman a small sum, Laura shakes her head, still feeling weak, as well as angry at herself for putting up with that. *What was I thinking? I should have walked out right away. That was no doctor . . . that was (thinking of the woman wearing a robe in the waiting room) like tribal medicine. Ancient, tribal Indian medicine. Old stuff.*

As she stands on the corner, she forgets which direction to go to return to the hotel. She feels a strong urge to call the American embassy or look up the nearest *real* doctor. She starts walking, and soon realizes this is not the right way back to the hotel. But just as she is about to turn around, she sees a small building painted in white, with a red cross on the front by the front door and the familiar staff-and-serpent symbol of the kind of medicine she is familiar with. She breathes in with a great sense of relief and walks over, re-energized, to the clinic. This time, everything looks much more familiar. A waiting room. What appears to be a nurse behind a desk. Clean chairs with magazines neatly arranged on a side table. A slight aroma of antiseptic.

The nurse says something in a language she cannot understand, and Laura looks at her and asks "English?" The nurse nods. "Yes, can I help you?"

The familiar phrase, the antiseptic smell, the familiar surroundings. It all feels comforting. She explains her situation to the nurse, sits down in a chair, closes

her eyes, and lets her body relax into the slightly frayed upholstery. In a few minutes, as expected, the nurse calls out "Laura Smith?" She is ushered into a small office where she notices the items that, in her mind, *ought* to be there—the scale, a blood pressure monitor, a stethoscope hanging on the wall. The equipment is a little old and worn, but at least it looks right. The nurse, efficiently takes her vital signs and temperature, then leaves the room.

About 10 minutes later, a woman in a white coat walks in. In halting English, looking at a form, she says "Yes . . . I see that you have a temperature. Your other vital signs are acceptable. Now, have you eaten anything in the past 2 days that . . . was . . . perhaps, not right? Had a smell that was not right?"

"No, I don't think so. Well not that I can remember."

"Have you been around anyone who was sick that you know of?"

Laura shakes her head.

"Have you been in any crowded places for a time . . . not a short time?"

Laura tries to remember. "No, except the bus station and the airport."

The doctor seems uncomfortable as she asks the next question. "Have you, well, I am sorry to ask, have you had many alcohol drinks in the past few nights?"

Laura shakes her head.

"Anything with drugs, you know, putting some in your body?"

Laura replies emphatically. "No, not at all."

"Does your throat hurt?"

"No, not really."

"Well you may have a virus, though I am not sure right now. I will prescribe two things for you—a pain reliever and something to calm your stomach and stop the vomiting if you keep doing that. I would like you to check back with me at the end of the day tomorrow. Please do not eat any fancy or rich food, just hot soup or things that are very simple with no spices. And rest. There is a pharmacy next door to this clinic. It is small but they will have these things. You may go now, and please see the nurse at the desk before you go."

"Thank you." Laura nods. This is more or less what she expects. She walks back out and the nurse tells her

FIGURE 1-2 Typical Waiting Room

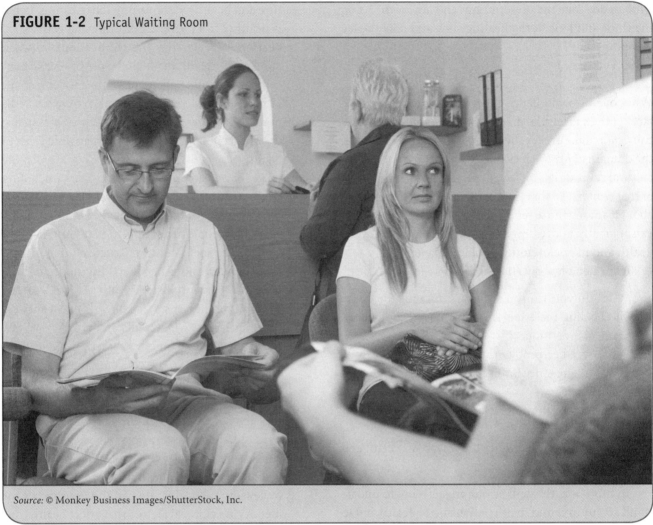

Source: © Monkey Business Images/ShutterStock, Inc.

that the charge will be 25 American dollars for the visit. She pays, and goes next door to buy the prescriptions recommended by the doctor.

With a few questions, she is able to re-orient her directions and walk slowly back to the hotel, which—*thankfully*—is only a few blocks away.

In her room, she sits down on her bed and tries to make sense of the day. *I mean, who was that healer? Wow, I sure didn't know what that was about. Should I just throw that stuff away that he gave me? I mean, I do have a prescription now. And what was all that he said to me about seasons and balances and all that? But, well, it was kind of interesting. All the stuff about too much hot seasons—in a way I kind of get what he meant by that.*

For the moment, she doesn't throw out the bag of healing materials he gave her, and tries to think about

FIGURE 1-3 Pills (Biomedical Magic)

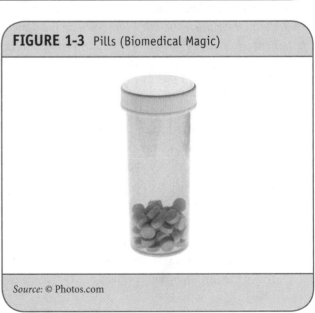

Source: © Photos.com

what to do. Take the prescriptions and lay down? Sit on the floor and look at the healing stick and take the tea and powder?

* * *

What our fictional Laura experiences is just one small facet of the substantial diversity that surrounds what we call *health*. Like every other domain of human existence, the domain of *health* does not exist apart from its socio-cultural context. It is, in fact, woven deeply into the fabric of that context, so that if we are to understand anything about it among the diversity of peoples and societies that exist globally, addressing the interconnections between health and its socio-cultural context is vital.

Consider a few questions:

1. What do you think Laura will do with the herbs and healing materials she got from the indigenous medical practitioner?
2. What was her problem with the setting and procedures she encountered with the indigenous practitioner?
3. Why do you think she felt more comfortable when she found a clinic?
4. What does her experience tell you about health and culture?

In this book, this will be our project—not to understand all cultures and their relationship to health, but to understand *how to think about that relationship, and how to work with the culture–health relationship in the design, implementation, and evaluation of health promotion efforts*. To do that, we will cover the following:

- After the introductory scenario about Laura Smith, Section One begins by introducing the concept of culture, not only through the analysis of definitions and specific features, but by presenting the idea in a broad sense as a key aspect of what makes us human. Culture will be connected to the way all humans interpret and make sense of life, to the way we are socially organized and carry out our daily tasks, and as a key source of motivation for behavior. Following this introduction, Section One draws the initial, broad connections between cul-

ture and health by examining the question, "what is health?" from several cultural perspectives.
- Section Two clarifies the connections between culture and health through the use of several conceptual tools and approaches—the idea of systems of health knowledge and practice known as ethnomedical systems and ethnopsychiatric systems; the connections between such systems and types of health treatments, as well as types of healers; the moral dimension of health and illness (including stigma) that flows from cultural views related to illness causation; the idea that vulnerability to disease (and people's reactions to that vulnerability) is shaped by socio-cultural structures that include class, gender, and other social divisions; and the idea that perceptions of health risk are filtered through cultural lenses that offer different answers to the question, "what is a health risk?"
- In Section Three, we move to practical applications and implications of the conceptual tools covered in Section Two. First, we take an in-depth look at several examples of health issues that are significantly impacted by cultural factors: HIV/AIDS, obesity and its consequences (diabetes, cardiovascular health), and youth violence—now viewed globally as a public health issue. Then there is a review of practical strategies and approaches for identifying cultural factors that affect health conditions, and working with these factors to develop and implement public health interventions that make sense in context and are more likely to be effective. These research strategies are followed by examples of health promotion programs that address a range of cultural factors. Finally, Section Three wraps up with a discussion of cultural competence—the way in which this term has been applied in relation to general efforts to eliminate disparities in health, and introducing a set of cultural competence principles that follow from the material covered in the book.

The general flow of these sections is intended to cover a continuum from understanding to action. After that, it's your turn!

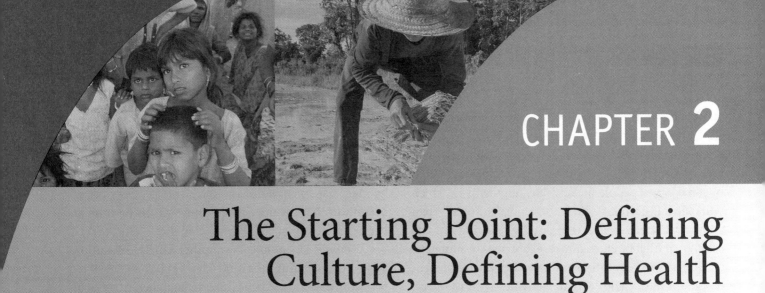

CHAPTER 2

The Starting Point: Defining Culture, Defining Health

"Humans cannot eat, breathe, defecate, mate, re-produce, sit, move about, sleep or lie down with-out following or expressing some aspect of their society's culture. Our cultures grow, expand, evolve. It's their nature."

—Marvin Harris

WHAT DO WE MEAN BY CULTURE?

Before proceeding any further, it is important to come to an understanding about what we mean by *culture*. After all, unless we arrive at a consensus about that, it will be difficult to carry on a discussion about culture and health. And it will be difficult to understand one of the fundamental bases for social behavior and diversity among human beings, as well as diversity in understandings and behaviors related to health. This, however, is not so easily done. Culture is one of those concepts that most people seem to intuitively grasp, yet cannot define clearly. It is probably the case that most people grasp it through the experience of *differences* in the way people look, act, talk, and carry out their daily lives that are more than individual differences, but seem to be common to some group of people that is distinct from one's own group. In these stereotype versions, dif-ferences come out in statements like:

- "English people are dour—they just never seem to laugh."
- "People from Latin American countries talk with their hands."
- "People from the islands are never in a hurry, they just take their time."

Whatever is or is not true about these stereotypes, they do not begin to touch the depth and complexity of what is included in the concept of culture. They are fleet-ing snapshots, highly biased by the observer's own defi-nition of what, for example, is funny, or how to behave when having a conversation, or what is or is not being in a hurry. Yet for many people they can represent some-thing significant about the way some group of people are. And though one group of people may not realize it when they have in mind a stereotype about another social or cultural group, the likelihood is that group also has re-ciprocal stereotypes. This process of categorizing groups of people as *others* (other than one's own group) is a com-mon feature of the way human beings think, and it forms a part of the whole phenomenon we think of as culture. But—whether in a public health or other context—as the world becomes more integrated and interdependent, it becomes ever more necessary to recognize the problems and limitations of such perceptions. We are all *others*, and it is important to develop the knowledge, skills, and understanding to cross these bridges.

There are other uses of the term *culture* that can confuse the situation. For example, if someone is said to be *cultured*, it doesn't have much to do with whether or not he/she is English, Guatemalan, or Tongan (though in some cases, people make value judgments in which one cultural group is said to be more "cultured" than another). Usually by that term, we are referring to some concept of high or elite culture, expressed through personal manners, education and knowledge, involvement in or familiarity with artistic activities such as opera, modern art, calligraphy, dance, or theater—that is contrasted to popular culture.

It should already be clear that what we are talking about in this chapter is not always easy to grasp or define. In fact, anthropologists who study human culture have been arguing about it for years, even though the culture concept is the central focus of study!

Definitions

In this book, we won't spend too much time on the specifics of one definition vs. another, because there are commonalities that are important. And certainly, questions about shared vs. unique characteristics of human societies go back a long way in the history of human inquiry. In the 5th century BCE, Greek historian Herodotus provided careful descriptions of peoples he encountered while chronicling the history of the Persian Wars. Fourteenth century (ACE) Arab historian and social philosopher Ibn Khaldun remains widely recognized for his insightful observations on social institutions and civilizations. The European political philosopher Jean Jacques Rousseau contrasted a universal, presocietal state of nature and the formation of civil societies, which, he argued, led to human difference and inequality. German philosopher J.G. Herder posited the idea of a historically evolved, integrated *bildung* (a collective identity) as a feature of humankind—a precursor to the theoretical construct of culture that emerged in the late 19th century.

The Classic Definition. As a starting point, let's take a look at a few of the more famous definitions of culture or at least types of definitions that have emerged from the field of cultural anthropology—the study of culture. The classic definition is an old but comprehensive one, from anthropologist E.B. Tylor in 1871 (Tylor 1871, pp.1; also see Kroeber & Kluckhohn's 1952 collection of culture definitions, 81), in which culture is said to be "that complex whole which includes knowledge, belief, art, morals, custom, and any other capabilities and habits acquired by man[1] as a member of society." This is a very broad definition that includes just about everything human connected to our socially connected life.

Symbolic Definition. Yet another kind of definition views human culture as a kind of symbolic text, in which behavior, objects, and belief interact together in a kind of ongoing dramatic production that represents issues and concepts of meaning for a particular society or group. Members of a culture act as characters in this grand drama, and what goes on (the plot) only makes sense in reference to an underlying interpretive framework. Clifford Geertz, a founder of what became known as symbolic anthropology, said, "Man is an animal suspended in webs of significance he himself has spun. I take culture to be those webs, and the analysis of it to be therefore not an experimental science in search of law but an interpretative one in search of meaning" (Geertz 1973, 5). But he also called it "an historically transmitted pattern of meanings embodied in symbols, a system of inherited conceptions expressed in symbolic forms by means of which men communicate, perpetuate, and develop their knowledge about and attitudes toward life" (Geertz 1973, 89). Victor Turner (1967, 1974), another seminal symbolic anthropologist, was well known for his study (among the Ndembu in Zambia) of rituals as symbolic productions in which the meaning of passage from one life stage to another was imparted through ritual elements, and the "liminal" period between one stage and another was characterized by a suspension of cultural rules and social roles.

Culture as Ideology. Still other, contemporary definitions of culture equate the concept to a kind of dominant *ideology* (following Gramsci 1971), or to beliefs, social institutions, practices, and media representations associated with particular configurations of power (e.g., Foucault 1972, 1980; Singer & Baer 1995; Singer 1997; Wolf 1982). For Michel Foucault, power takes its effect through discourse, the various and related forms of language and representation that characterize a particular historical

---

[1] This was the late 19th century, hence the use of *man*.

period. Discourse at any point with a configuration of power, and the "rules" for interpreting what is or is not a valid statement. According to this view, in modern, industrial-capitalist Western culture, where health and health care are market commodities, the prevailing discourse would objectivize disease into discrete, analytical categories that, in the grand scheme of things, are easily tied to specific treatments and medications—all of which fits neatly into a product framework.

Cultural Materialist Definitions. Another approach views culture primarily as a *system of belief, practice, and technology directly tied to economic activity or to the adaptation of a people to a particular physical environment.* Cultural theory of this type has been called economic, ecological, or materialist anthropology. The anthropologist Marvin Harris famously argued, for example, that the veneration of cattle among Hindu peoples was a cultural belief that grew out of the centrality of cattle to the Indian diet (e.g., meat, milk) and food production system (Harris 1966). Julian Steward, an ecological anthropologist, theorized the existence of *culture cores* (patterns of social organization, technology, etc.) that should be the same wherever there was a similar physical environment (Steward 1955). Roy Rappaport (1984, 223) said that culture is ". . . a part of the distinctive means by which a local population maintains itself in an ecosystem and by which a regional population maintains and coordinates its groups and distributes them over the available land."

Linguistic Definition. You can also think of culture as a kind of *language.* Speakers of the language may use it differently, to create slang, irony, humor, or even poetry. Or they may break the rules to create a particular effect, but it's the same language, and underneath that language is some shared base of understanding about the nature of existence and day-to-day life. Try looking sometime at a transcript of a conversation between two people (from the same society or culture). You will often see that many sentences are left unfinished. Why? Because it is not necessary to finish them, since both conversants know the underlying information that makes the conversation possible. The conversation becomes a kind of exercise in reference points.

Mental or Cognitive Definitions. A different kind of definition constructs culture as something primarily *in the mind* of people within a particular group, a kind of shared conceptual framework that organizes thought and behavior. From this perspective, culture is not so much about what people do, but about what they think and how that determines what they do. One of the earliest and most widely known of these definitions, from Ward Goodenough, states that culture "consists of whatever it is one has to know or believe in order to operate in a manner acceptable to its members" (Goodenough 1957, pp. 167). Related to this is the idea of culture as a complex, shared (more or less) set of models or schema, at many levels, that enable people to interpret situations and then feel and act appropriately—that is, within a range that would make sense to others who also shared those models. Cultural models theory (see D'Andrade & Strauss 1992; Holland & Quinn 1987; Holland et al. 1998; Shore 1996) posits interacting models at many levels, for the day to day, in the form of behavioral "scripts" (e.g., a script for the proper way to introduce yourself to your fiancee's family), to higher level models for gender, family, and the progression of life.

Still another cognitive conceptualization of culture uses the information processing analogy of a software program—though one should not go too far with this because it can make the idea of culture appear mechanistic. Software programs include many default settings and automatic operations that serve as shortcuts so that the system as a whole can do its job more quickly and efficiently. In a sense, culture operates the same way. In everyday life, if you were constantly faced with situations at many levels which you knew nothing about and didn't know how to interpret or react to, how would you act? Instead, over time, common patterns of thought and behavior become part of the shared corpus (culture) that no longer needs to be thought about actively, creating a situation in which people in that culture often use default settings or shortcuts concerning those background facts in order to facilitate the management of everyday life.

Cultural and Biocultural. Finally (for now), and especially in the context of public health, yet another way to think of culture in relation to the human condition is to understand human beings as *biocultural.* We are, without a doubt, biological beings, consisting of physical, chemical, and other biological processes. But we have a unique ability to interpret our biological selves in

EXHIBIT 2-1   An Example: The Classroom as Cultural Construct

We can illustrate this by using a classroom as an example. Think about it this way: When you walk into a classroom, without thinking about it, you already know what the typical classroom setup is, with students sitting at desks, and an instructor or professor up front. The professor lectures; students take notes. You already know what kinds of clothing are appropriate to wear in a classroom. You have an expectation about the kind of behavior that is appropriate (you wouldn't, after all, scream, do handstands, or wriggle on the floor for no reason). You have in mind the type of people who are generally in a classroom. Importantly, you already understand the role a classroom plays in the social setting you call "college," and you know what role a classroom plays in getting a degree, and in turn what role getting a degree is likely to have on your future job and social prospects. All this you know without thinking about it at all—because all of this knowledge is essentially a default setting, based on what is known as a cultural model or schema for classroom.

Now suppose you didn't know any of this. You had no cultural model for classroom. But for some reason, you were placed in a classroom by some well-meaning soul who wanted to expose you to these things. Let's say you had been brought up in a prison, and had never attended, seen, heard about, or experienced a classroom. What you do see when you walk in to that classroom are four walls (no windows), and a lot of people crowded together and sitting down. Without thinking, you connect what you are seeing to the nearest cultural model you have, which comes form your prison upbringing. Your default settings kick in. You are in a confined space, like prison. There are a lot of people, and they can all see you. Your first thought is that there is danger in this situation, and you will have to assert yourself right away to establish a reputation necessary to protect yourself. As you walk down the aisle, a student accidentally drops her purse on the floor in front of you, causing you to stumble slightly. Immediately, your stomach tightens. Your eyes rove back and forth to gauge who has seen this blatant act of disrespect. With barely a thought, almost as if automatic, you know that you have to make it clear in a big way that no one will be allowed to disrespect you like that. You turn and start pummeling the student hard with your fists. The other students are horrified, and one runs outside to get security. Two security guards rush in and pin you down. But you are secure in the knowledge that, when you are back in this room, the others will know what to expect from you and will be reluctant to harm you.

The students think you are crazy. You have no idea that they do, and wouldn't understand why. Two different models and default settings are at work, both legitimate. Both lead to different interpretations of what the situation is, and thus to different behaviors

---

many ways and to put a particular kind of stamp on the biological world in which we live. What to one group of people would be a willingness to accept senseless pain is to another a praiseworthy example of self-sacrifice and religious purity. Or take the example of hunger. This is clearly a biological phenomenon—when our bodies need food, we are hungry. But it also intersects with a very nonbiologic phenomenon; the cultural process of categorizing food as edible or not edible. In theory, anything that provides nutrition and is not poisonous should be edible. But that isn't the case. Would you eat a cockroach raw, if presented to you right now? Would you eat a dog or a cat? Would you eat the eyes from an animal you are eating? Do you eat meat? It is only when human beings are starving (or on a reality television show perhaps?) that the biological imperatives take over and people may forgo their cultural categorizations.

These are all beliefs and behaviors related to food that follow from an interpretation of the biological world, a system of categorization (with justifications) that deems some things edible and others not. But as you can see, this is not biological. It is not a given. It is something that it is imposed on the biological world by a society or group of people who have, over many years, developed a system of beliefs and practices about food and eating. Some people within that culture will adhere rigidly to these ideas, maybe even when they are starving. Others will not, and may experiment. But in either case, it is possible to look at that integrated set of beliefs and practices and understand it as something cultural, that interacts with the biological. Scholars of culture, including Mary Douglas (1966), Claude Levi-Strauss (1969), and others have long been interested in the way culture—as a human phenomenon—often involves deep systems of categorization in which the things of the world are divided into such groupings as pure vs. polluted, male vs. female, hot vs. cold, or, as we have noted, edible vs. not edible. In this book, we will see this process as applied to health.

Without going on for pages and pages about this, consider that most definitions of culture share the following basic components, to one degree or another: (1) it is a phenomenon that exists as a kind of whole—that is, an integrated pattern of some kind, which links together many aspects of life and social structure within a group or society; (2) it refers to the relationship between what people know and believe, and what they do; (3) it is acquired—that is, you are not born with it, but you learn it during the course of life in society; and (4) it is shared, more or less, among members of the group or society, and transmitted to members of the group/society over time. On the latter point, the concept of culture—because it refers to a general human characteristics—is applicable to many types of social groups and structures that exist over time, from societies as a whole, to regional and tribal groups, or to smaller subgroups that could include anything from gangs to workplaces.

You can see that there is a lot of room for clarification, even in these four basic points. For example, what do we mean by saying that culture is an integrated pattern? This is not an either-or statement—nothing is perfectly integrated vs. completely nonintegrated. What is meant here, and this will become very important in our later discussions of culture and health, is that culture refers in part to a human tendency for *coherence*, so that the way we live "hangs together" and makes sense in some way. Let's take just one situation. Many times in the news you hear references to democracy, and whether or not a political process, in the United States or in another country, is democratic. Think about that for a moment. What does it mean to be democratic, and how should we judge whether something is or isn't? Usually, we make this judgment starting from a general idea like, "democracy means rule by the people." We may then get more specific, saying that there should be elections, a constitution, and a multiparty legislature to make laws. But all of these specific manifestations of democracy depend not only on a particular history, but on a cultural belief about the nature of individuals in relation to the state or governing body. That is what makes these specific activities hang together. If you are from a culture in which individuals are thought of primarily as representatives of a clan, or a village—more so than as individuals—then elections where individuals vote may not be understood the same way as they would be understood in Anglo-American or Western culture. People might simply vote as a clan, or a village, and it might not seem odd at all for other members of the clan or village to ask you if you voted the right way.

Furthermore, they would think of that as normal, *natural*—because much of what we believe as a result of cultural learning drops below the conscious radar and seems to be *the way it is*, not worth thinking about.

And consider the idea of culture as something shared among a group of people. This is a very important part of the idea of culture. Yet in any society or group, not everyone shares one single set of precise cultural beliefs and behaviors. Some people disagree with others about certain issues or rules. Different expectations about behavior may apply to some subgroups more than others. People who share a culture may also incorporate beliefs or practices from another culture, or more than one. So why do we think of it as shared? Because, first of all, no culture is ironclad or fixed. Cultures always change,

BOX 2-1 Do Only Human Beings Have Culture?

If we think of culture primarily as learned behavior, than are humans the only species that has culture and can transmit it? A number of other species have been shown to transmit or teach behaviors to others in the same species. For example, many higher primates (e.g., chimpanzees and orangutans) teach their young to use simple tools such as a stick to probe for termites or leafy branches to draw water from a hole.

But is this culture? Probably not. Culture is much more than learned behavior. It involves learned behavior as a part of a system of meaning, interpretation, and action that is communicated through language, symbolized through various forms of representation, integrated with social and economic structures, and transmitted among groups and societies over time.

adapt, and evolve over time. But more important, what we think of as culture is necessarily a kind of fluid, open construct—more like a central tendency or home base, or a tool kit for how to live. Moreover, if you examine most disagreements or conflicts within a culture, they are not conflicts about culture as a whole, but about interpretations of cultural elements. To use the example of democracy again, people from Anglo-American culture may argue about whether or not a specific type of election is really democratic or not, but they are most likely operating from the same basic belief structure about the role of individuals and simply disagree on whether or not a type of election adheres to that belief. This is a very different kind of argument than would occur between a person who shared that idea of individualism and one who believed that individuals were not the primary unit in society.

Related to the issue of sharing culture is the problem of *boundaries*. How can we define the people who share a particular culture? Is it a political definition—people from one country share one culture? In most cases, clearly not. Is it another kind of geographic boundary, such as a region (itself defined by some feature like mountains, or a valley, or a river)? Or is it a social boundary, like class, where people of a certain class are said to share a culture (in this case, perhaps an ideological component as well)? Is it religion? Now that is an interesting case, for if you look at major religions that are globally diffused, you will often find that people in different locations who nominally share the same religion practice a different version of that religion, typically influenced by local culture.[2] Or is it related to interest groups—where, for example, people who are avid bicyclists can be said to share a culture? The truth is, culture as it exists in the world may include some aspects of all of these boundaries. Moreover, culture is not fixed but evolves, as people from one society or group come into contact with other people, or as they change over time, their cultures change. Add to that the deep and ubiquitous influence of electronic media (Internet, mobile technologies, television, film, etc.), through which the symbols, stories, beliefs and practices of any one culture may be influenced by others and diffused among many others.

The boundary problem also lies within any culture. When one society includes diverse groups, either based on class, region, ethnicity, gender, or another characteristic, what can we say about that society's culture? Is there some kind of culture *core* to look for? Who determines the culture of that society? This has been a major issue of focus among scholars of culture, who have examined the way in which diverse cultures or diverse cultural elements within one political unit such as a state are sometimes controlled and shaped by those who have the power to do so—via control over economic resources, media, political control, or dominant influence over the social structure. This leads to the question, "whose cul-

---

EXHIBIT 2-2 Culture and the Body

One day, I was observing a dance class at a Buddhist temple primarily attended by Southeast Asian immigrants in the United States. The class was for girls and young women and led by a very serious-looking older woman who was highly skilled, leading the class through a specific dance that they were to perform at an upcoming festival. Her movements were graceful and precise, enacted as if every extended motion of her hands and extension of her leg was of great consequence, as if each move were like the turning of the earth itself around its axis.

The girls in the class seemed to have picked up her sense of the importance of these movements, and with all earnestness they moved through the steps, bobbing up and down, turning one foot one way, then another at a set angle, extending one arm and hand out like a branch of a young sapling, as their other hand clutched a bouquet of flowers.

It struck me, as an observer, that in this coordinated series of movements, there was a lesson involved, a cultural lesson, and a gender lesson. And it was a lesson learned not by words, stories, or rules, but by training the girls in a culturally shaped sense of physical being. That lesson may have had to do with how to physically relate to the world around oneself, with grace, with restraint, and in so doing symbolically portraying a female gendered *modus vivendi*, what Pierre Bourdieu has referred to as a "bodily hexis" (1977). It is very likely that this particular bodily sensibility is mirrored in other cultural discourse surrounding female gender qualities.

---

[2] The term for such blending is *syncretic*.

ture?" when drawing conclusions or making statements about a particular society. In such cases, to understand the cultural landscape of any given society means some examination of the competing, conflicting, coexisting, and consensus cultures within it.

Culture, Subcultures, and Other Structures of Diversity. Before we move on, it is important to touch on the way the concept of culture is also used in reference to groups that are smaller than whole societies or populations—sometimes a lot smaller. Again, because having culture is simply a part of the human makeup, whenever there is a group of some kind that is sustained for a reasonable period of time, it is likely that shared patterns of behavior and attitude will develop. That is key to human diversity. Here we could be referring to people who play rugby, to punk rock musicians, to southerners or northerners (region), to corporate cultures, or to more fundamental groupings like gender or people who are of a similar socioeconomic or class background. In order to analyze the latter, sociologist Pierre Bourdieu (1977) came up with the concept of a *habitus*, which generally refers to patterns of behavior, social relations, discourse, attitudes, styles, and social expectations associated with people who share a particular socioeconomic circumstance. Some cultural patterns—often referred to as "pop culture"—seem to be connected to specific age groups, and while they are sustained for a while, they dissipate or are diffused into broader cultural practices.

WHAT DO WE MEAN BY HEALTH?

Now that we have some ideas about the concept of culture, it is time to move toward making the connection between culture and health. First, we have to decide what we mean by health. That should be obvious, right? Not necessarily. There are several ways to think about what the term *health* means. One is based on strictly biomedical criteria. So, for example, if you say "John is healthy," by this standard you might mean:

- John is free of disease (i.e., no pathogens have overcome his immune system and caused physical symptoms).
- John's body functions normally (his organs, vascular, nervous, and other systems function as they should).

- John is free of injury or physical problems.
- John eats healthy food (food that provides essential nutrients and is free of substances that cause damage to bodily functions).
- John engages in healthy, preventive behaviors (e.g., brushing teeth, basic hygiene, immunizations, visiting doctors).
- John avoids behaviors that are health risks.
- John is in reasonable physical shape.

But let's go a little further. When people say, "John is healthy," they may also mean:

- John looks happy.
- John is satisfied with his life.
- John gets along with people.
- John looks good.
- John dresses well.
- John is liked by others.

Or even . . .

- John is doing well (meaning, he has a decent income, a good car, etc.).
- John connects with the spiritual world.
- John has good relations with his extended family, as well as his ancestors.

So there is often more going on here than just biomedical health. From these statements, there also seems to be an element of mental health, general well-being, social relations, and socioeconomic status. The World Health Organization, part of the United Nations, defines health as "a state of complete physical, mental and social well-being and not merely the absence of infirmity" (WHO 1948, pp. 1). This implies that to be healthy, people should be living in decent conditions, with basic needs met.

If you examine what people mean by *healthy* across many cultures, you will encounter other criteria. Some of these criteria might even conflict with biomedical standards. For example, in many parts of the world, when someone is large—what might be called "obese"—this is viewed as evidence of material well-being, or in the case of females, fertility, maternal capability, or warm personality. So in that culture, if people are asked whether or not John is healthy (remember that he is in good physical shape), they might say "Well, he is a little thin. He must not be eating well. Or maybe he doesn't have enough to eat." And if he doesn't have enough to eat, it might mean he doesn't have a good enough social position.

Or take the idea that a healthy John avoids behaviors that are health risks. But in some cultures, people are admired for taking certain kinds of risks. It may even be necessary. Most cultures include ideas about passing from one stage of life to another, and the movements between stages are typically marked by a ritual, known as a *rite of passage*. Sometimes such rituals involve an element of risk. At one time, young Maasai men in Kenya were supposed to fight with a lion as a rite of passage, to prove their bravery (Maasai Association). Among some American Indian peoples, young men had to go off by

themselves for a period of days in the wilderness, without eating, in order to have a vision experience, as a requirement for moving on to manhood (see, for example, Powers 1982). These rites often involve what we might call "health risks," yet they are understood to be good and absolutely necessary to proceed to the next life stage. In the United States, drinking alcohol has sometimes been viewed by young people as a rite of passage, which may have something to do with the emotions tied up in underage drinking, the willingness to engage in very risky behaviors connected to drinking, and the way in which alcohol-related escapades are related in next-day tales with a certain amount of relish.

Health as Being Well, However Defined. The message here is that to understand diverse concepts of health and

FIGURE 2-1 American Indian/Alaska Native Youth—Health as a Community Construct

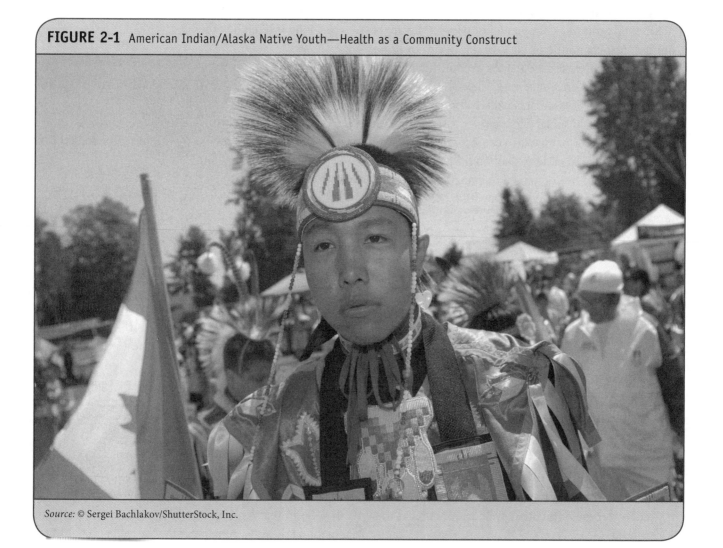

Source: © Sergei Bachlakov/ShutterStock, Inc.

healthy behavior, it is necessary to think of health in a broader way, beyond the biomedical. Health, for a given culture, is often very close to ideas within that culture about being well. So, for this book and as a reminder to think about health cross-culturally, *we will think of being healthy as synonymous with being well, however defined. That also means that being unhealthy can be seen as not being well, however that is defined.*

Let's look at some definitions and descriptions across cultures concerning what it means to be healthy, noting that in Western cultures, being healthy has often referred simply to the absence of disease (Galanti 2004).

North American Indian/First Nation Peoples. Many North American Indian peoples in the United States and Canada (sometimes referred to as First Nations) think of being healthy in terms of a balance represented in what is called the "medicine wheel" (see Whiskey-jack, n.d.), which includes mental, physical, emotional and spiritual components within a holistic definition of being healthy (see Isaak & Marchessault 2008 and Turton 1997). "The interconnectedness of the quadrants in the wheel represent the relationship of the individual with his or her family, his or her community, and the world, and balancing each aspect of the wheel is considered to be crucial for optimal growth and development" (Isaak & Marchessault 2008, 115). In a study done with adults and youth who were members of the Manitoba Cree people (ibid.), many of the study respondents said that health to them was not just the absence of physical illness. Someone could have no physical problems and still not be considered healthy. In addition, some respondents in this study reiterated the idea that for the Manitoba Cree (as for other American Indian groups), health is not an individual construct, but a collective one—that is, individuals are not fully healthy unless the community is healthy.

Native Hawaiians. According to some accounts (McMullin 2005), Native Hawaiian constructs of health do not focus on health as an attribute of individuals. Instead, it is tied to maintaining Hawaiian culture in the face of social and historical relations that have marginalized that culture. In other words, "health" means "being Hawaiian" in the way that Hawaiians used to be. Much like the situation for American Indians, the decline in health for native Hawaiians (currently experiencing high rates of diabetes, cardiovascular disease, and other problems) occurred as a direct result of colonization, including disease for which Hawaiians had no immunity or previous exposure, as well as appropriation and privatization of Hawaiian land which in turn limited access to traditional agricultural foods and fish. So, returning to traditional identity would be synonymous with eating more fish, shrimp and plant foods such as taro, poi (from taro), and hihiawai (edible fern), which, of course, are healthier foods than many now available to Hawaiians. Like many American Indian peoples, Hawaiian ideas of health—referred to as "lokahi"—are not confined to

FIGURE 2-2 Native Hawaiians—Health as Identity

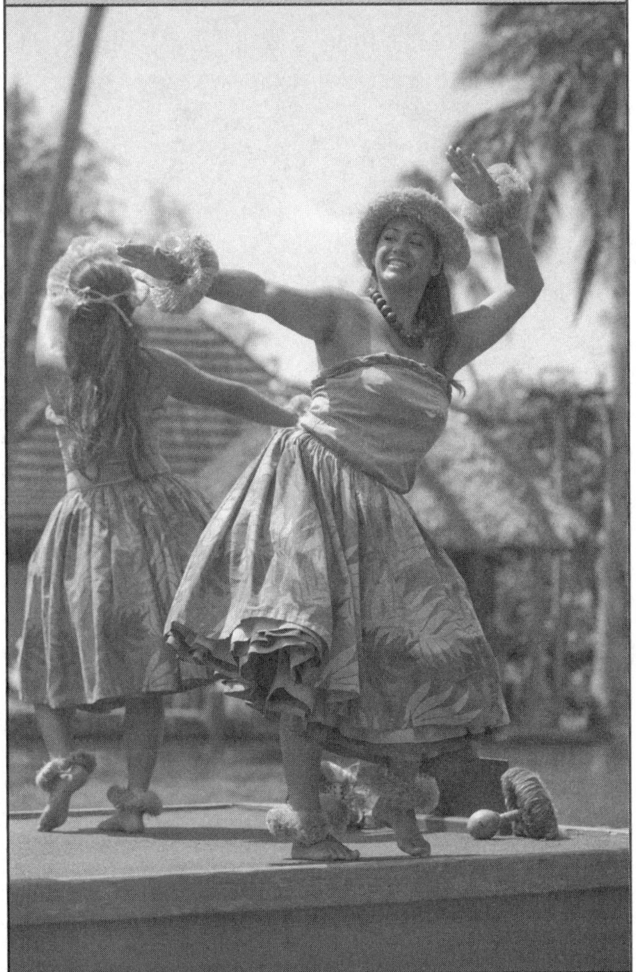

Source: © Jose Gil/ShutterStock, Inc.

physical health, but involve a balance or harmony between all aspects of life. In addition, some respondents in the study conducted by McMullin (ibid.) equated being healthy with practicing Hawaiian culture.

Urban Senegalese Women. As noted previously, a number of studies have shown that, in non-Western cultures, large body size for women is associated with multiple dimensions of what people refer to as health. One study in Senegal (West Africa) with about 300 women ages 20–50 (Holdsworth et al. 2004) used an interesting approach to get at the meaning of body size. Women in the study were shown a set of body silhouettes, ranging from very thin to obese based on their correspondence to body mass index, the biomedical standard used for assessing healthy body weight. The women were asked

to comment about what those profiles represented. The silhouettes showing overweight women were linked to a range of positive personal attributes—warm, happy, popular, friendly, proud, sociable, easy going, and having a strong personality. Body size profiles leaning towards the overweight were also seen as having the highest social status, a good job, enough money, a contented husband, children, proud family in-laws, and a higher likelihood of getting married. In contrast to similar studies and possibly due to increasing Western influence, some positive attributes were also assigned to biomedically normative body size images, and the obese images were linked to negative characteristics. The highest positives were linked to the overweight profile—suggesting that such a profile was viewed by most of the women as *healthy.*

FIGURE 2-3 Being Healthy in Thailand—Harmony and Social Relationships

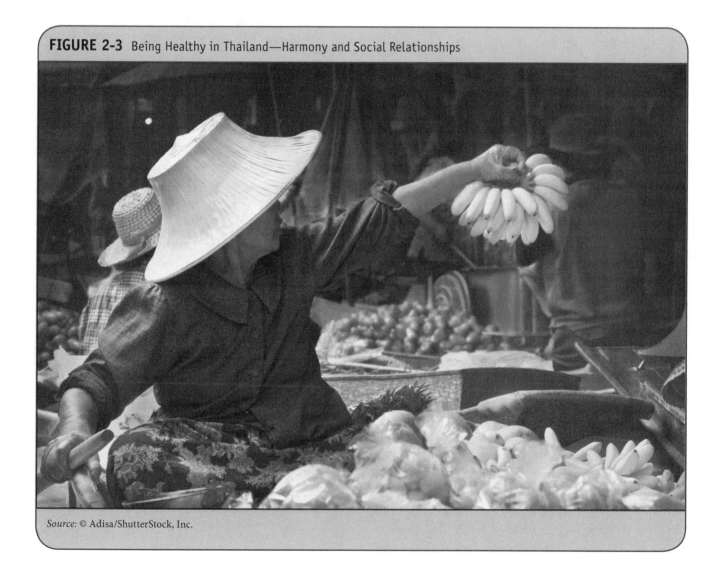

Source: © Adisa/ShutterStock, Inc.

Being Healthy in Thailand. In Thailand, which is a primarily Buddhist culture in which the idea of an individual self is viewed differently than it is in Western culture (see Markus & Kitayama 1998, 1994, 1991), the idea of health and well-being is tied to relations and interdependence with other people. Once again, in Thai culture health is not a solely individual construct. From interviews conducted with 67 healthy Thai older adults (Ingersoll-Dayton et al. 2001), one study concluded that well-being included five dimensions for these Thai elders: harmony, interdependence, acceptance, respect, and enjoyment. Harmony included family harmony, harmony in the families of one's children, and positive relations with neighbors and friends. Interdependence had a lot to do with family members helping each other—especially children helping adults as they got older (an important role for children). Acceptance referred to the very Buddhist stance of accepting what life brings in a calm state—in part because it is believed that what happens to a person in this life is a result of what he or she did in a previous life (the idea of karma). Respect referred to social standing and the age-related respect an adult should receive from children and those younger than they were. This is a very important aspect of proper social relations. Finally, the idea of enjoyment as part of well-being had to do with appreciating simple pleasures and the combination of fun with work.

Any way you look at it, health is a domain of culture, intertwined with the fabric of life and the beliefs and practices that go with it. Of importance, health and culture exist and interact within a broader social, political and economic environment. To fully understand any particular culture and its health domain, it is sometimes necessary to step back and take a look at the interaction between a society or group of people and its surrounding environment, as illustrated in Figure 2-4.

With that in mind, take a look at a particular subpopulation that has been at high risk for HIV/AIDS in the United States, particularly in urban areas—injection drug users who are African American.

If we break the situation down into levels of a social ecology, it might look like this:

- As processes internal to American culture, African Americans are a group that was incorporated into the larger population originally through slavery, and then through extensive de jure and de facto segregation, until very recently. Thus there are attitudes and practices about the social relationship of African Americans that are embedded in American culture and have resulted in a long history of exclusion and marginalization.
- The institution of slavery itself (in the Americas) developed as a result of the colonial exploitation of the land and mineral wealth of the Americas and Caribbean for European purposes. As an offspring of European culture, the evolving American culture also adopted and benefited from slavery, primarily in the Southern states.

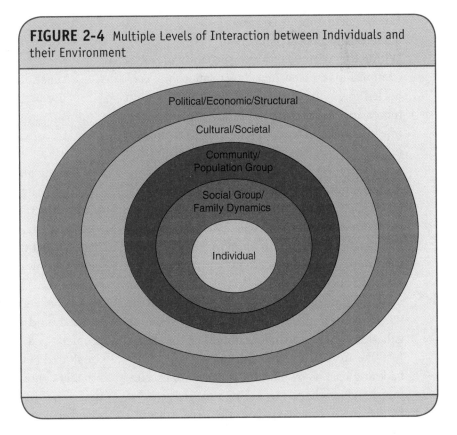

FIGURE 2-4 Multiple Levels of Interaction between Individuals and their Environment

Political/Economic/Structural

Cultural/Societal

Community/Population Group

Social Group/Family Dynamics

Individual

- It wasn't until the early and mid 20th century that African Americans migrated northward, seeking work in the burgeoning industrial economy. Because of cultural attitudes about race, most of these African Americans lived in specific concentrations within urban areas. By and large, even these African Americans were excluded from equal education and certainly better paying and more powerful job opportunities.

- African American industrial workers, while experiencing some economic gains, were still in a precarious position. They were particularly vulnerable to any industrial downturn and loss of jobs—which of course did occur during the Depression and much later after World War II when the northern industrial base began to diminish because of increasing global competition.

- Within these deindustrializing urban areas, social relationships evolved, including relationships connected to coping and survival strategies, within increasingly marginalized inner city areas that offered fewer and fewer opportunities for employment. One such pattern of social relationships and accompanying subculture, was integrally connected to underground economies based on illegal goods such as drugs and the ready market among people seeking ways to cope. The prevalence of drug use (e.g., heroin, cocaine) created its own subgroups—people whose lives centered on the acquisition and use of drugs. Part of this subculture included sharing of injection equipment, and the use of drugs in group settings such as "shooting galleries" (often in abandoned buildings or alleys). Just like any culture, the injection use subculture had (and has) its own attitudes, social roles, customs, and language—including a shared sense of its marginalized role vis-à-vis the larger society.

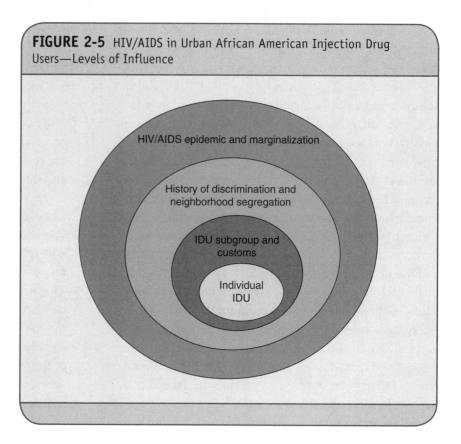

FIGURE 2-5 HIV/AIDS in Urban African American Injection Drug Users—Levels of Influence

- Soon after the HIV epidemic first hit, it spread into the injection drug user subpopulation in part because of customs related to sharing and the group use settings—and of course because the use of shared needles was a direct source of body fluid transmission.

Taking all these facts into account, the context for injection drug user subcultures and their relationship to the health crisis of HIV/AIDS begins to add up. Ideally, knowing this context, and having some understanding of injection drug user subculture(s) should help in determining useful approaches to prevention and intervention. The patterns of behavior, how they came about, beliefs, attitudes, social roles that exist—all of these should provide a foundation for addressing the problem as a human problem, as one that arises from the shared nature of all humans to create worlds within broader contexts. This is a way of understanding health issues that fits very much into the increasingly recognized ecological model in public health.

REFERENCES

Bourdieu, P. 1977. *Outline of a Theory of Practice*. Cambridge: Cambridge University Press.

D'Andrade, R., and C. Strauss, eds. 1992. *Human Motives and Cultural Models*. Cambridge: Cambridge University Press.

Douglas, M. 1966. *Purity & Danger: An Analysis of the Concepts of Pollution and Taboo*. London: Routledge & Kegan Paul.

Foucault, M. 1972. *The Archaeology of Knowledge*. Translated by A.M. Sheridan Smith. New York: Harper Colophon.

Foucault M. 1980. *Power/Knowledge: Selected Interviews and Other Writings, 1972–1977*. Edited by C. Gordon. Translated by C. Gordon, L. Marshall, J. Mepham, and K. Soper. New York: Pantheon Books.

Galanti, G.A. 2004. *Caring for Patients from Different Cultures*, 3rd ed. Philadelphia: University of Pennsylvania Press.

Geertz, C. 1973. *The Interpretation of Cultures: Selected Essays*. New York: Basic Books.

Goodenough, WH. 1957. "Cultural Anthropology and Linguisics." In PL Garvin (Ed), *Report of the Seventh Annual Rountable Meeting on Linguistics and Languiage Study*, p. 167-173. Washington, DC: Georgetown University Press.

Gramsci, A. 1971. *Selections from Prison Notebooks*. London: Lawrence and Wishart.

Harris, M. 1966. "The Cultural Ecology of India's Sacred Cattle." *Current Anthropology* 7 (1): 51–66.

Holdsworth, M., A. Gartner, E. Landais, B. Maire, and F. Delpeuch. 2004. "Perceptions of Healthy and Desirable Body Size in Urban Senegalese Women." *International Journal of Obesity* 28: 1561–1568.

Holland, D., W. Lachicotte, Jr., D. Skinner, and C. Cain. 1998. *Identity and Agency in Cultural Worlds*. Cambridge, MA; Harvard University Press.

Holland, D., and N. Quinn, eds. 1987. *Cultural Models in Language and Thought*. Cambridge: Cambridge University Press.

Ingersoll-Dayton, B., C. Saengtienchai, J. Kespichayawattana, and Y. Aungsuroch. 2001. "Psychological Well-Being Asian Style: The Perspective of Thai Elders." *Journal of Cross-Cultural Gerentology* 16: 283–302.

Isaak, C.A., and G. Marchessault. 2008. "Meaning of Health: The Perspectives of Aboriginal Adults and Youth in a Northern Manitoba First Nations Community." *Canadian Journal of Diabetes* 32 (2): 114–122.

Kroeber, A.L., and C. Kluckhohn. 1952. *Culture: A Critical Review of Concepts and Definitions*. New York: Vintage Books.

Levi-Strauss, C. 1969. *The Raw and the Cooked (Mythologiques Vol. 1)*. English translation, New York: Harper & Row.

Maasai Association website, accessed September 2010, www.maasai-association.org/lion.html.

Markus, H., and S. Kitayama. 1991. "Culture and the Self: Implications for Cognition, Emotion and Motivation." *Psychological Review* 98: 224–253.

Markus, H., and S. Kitayama. 1994. "The Cultural Construction of Self and Emotion: Implications for Social behavior." In *Emotion and Culture*, edited by S. Kitayama and H. Markus, 89–130. Washington, DC: American Psychological Association.

Markus, H., and S. Kitayama. 1998. "The Cultural Psychology of Personality." *Journal of Cross-Cultural Psychology* 29: 63–87.

McMullin, J. 2005. "The Call to Life: Revitalizing a Healthy Hawaiian Identity." *Social Science & Medicine* 61: 809–820.

Powers, W.K. 1982. *Yuwipi: Vision and Experience in Oglala Ritual*. Lincoln: University of Nebraska Press.

Rappaport, R.A. 1984. *Pigs for the Ancestors*, 2nd ed. New Haven, CT: Yale University Press.

Shore, B. 1996. *Culture in Mind: Cognition, Culture and the Problem of Meaning*. Oxford: Oxford University Press.

Singer, M., and H. Baer. 1995. *Critical Medical Anthropology*. Amityville, NY: Baywood Publishing Co.

Singer, M. (Ed.) 1997. *The Political Economy of AIDS*. Amityville, NY: Baywood Publishing Co.

Steward, J. 1955. *Theory of Culture Change: The Methodology of Multilinear Evolution*. Urbana: University of Illinois Press.

Turner, V. 1967. *The Forest of Symbols: Aspects of Ndembu Ritual*. Ithaca, NY: Cornell University Press.

Turner, V. 1974. *Dramas, Fields, and Metaphors: Symbolic Action in Human Society*. Ithaca, NY: Cornell University Press.

Turton, C.L. 1997. "Ways of Knowing About Health: An Aboriginal Perspective." *Annals of Advanced Nursing Science* 19: 28–36.

Tylor, E.B. 1871. *Primitive Culture*. 2 vols. New York: Brentano's.

Whiskeyjack, F., n.d. "The Medicine Wheel." Four Directions Teachings, Accessed September 2010. linna.ca/page8.html

WHO. 1948. Preamble to the Constitution of the World Health Organization, adopted by the International Health Conference, New York, 19–22 June, 1946; signed on 22 July 1946 by the representatives of 61 States (Official Records of the World Health Organization, no. 2, p. 100) and entered into force on April 7, 1948.

Wolf, E. 1982. *Europe and the People Without History*. Berkeley: University of California Press.

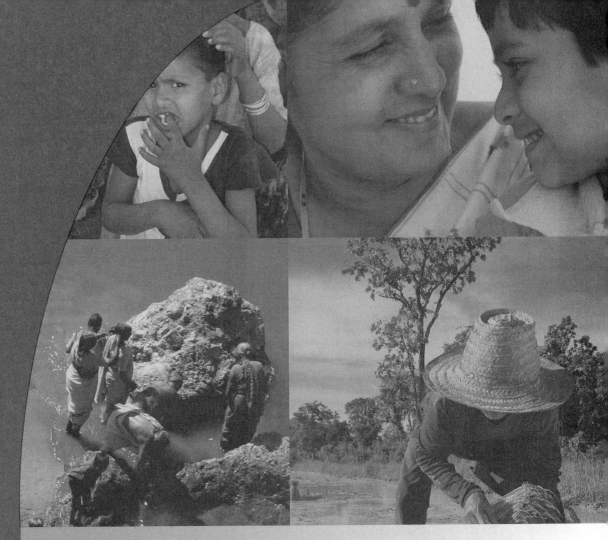

SECTION TWO

Tools and Perspectives for Understanding the Relationship between Culture and Health

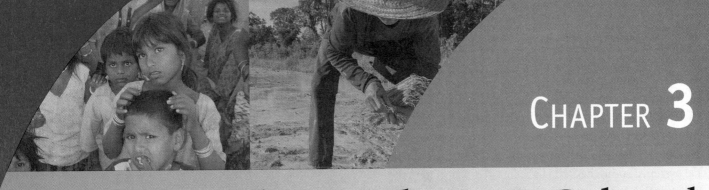

CHAPTER 3

Ethnomedicine I: Cultural Health Systems of Related Knowledge and Practice

"Every historic culture-pattern is an organic whole in which all the parts are interdependent."

—Historian Arnold Toynbee[1]

In Chapter 2, we reviewed different kinds of definitions of culture. One type of definition was a cognitive or mental definition—that is, culture is something that exists in the mind (as an interpretive system, as a system for processing information, or a model). The approach to linking culture and health we will review in this chapter draws from that perspective. Of course, even a cognitive definition of culture makes the connection between what people think and what they do, so what we are discussing here doesn't just exist in the mind, but is translated into action.

In Chapter 2, we also considered the example of a classroom as a cultural construct that shapes people's understandings about what to do and not do in the physical and social space called a "classroom." In a health context, a similar process is at work, though at a more basic level because we are not just talking about passing a class or getting a degree, but about key life issues of health and well-being. Also in Chapter 2, the idea of health as a cultural construct was linked to ideas about *being well* versus *not being well*. This is the starting point for think-

ing about the idea of an *ethnomedical system*, which is essentially a system of classification connected to a cultural definition of being well or not well. For this book, we will define an ethnomedical system as: *an applied cultural knowledge system related to health that sets out the kinds of health problems that can exist, their causes, and (based on their causes) appropriate treatments—as an interrelated system of belief and practice.*

It is, in an important way, a working understanding of health and treatment shared by a particular cultural group. It is like a cultural guidebook to the following questions:

- What can go wrong—or what are the signs and symptoms of not being well?
- Why do these things happen (cause)?
- What should someone do about it (treatment)?

Of key importance when thinking about the cultural aspect of ethnomedical systems is that, across cultures, there are different answers to all of these questions, from the range of potential health problems, to causes, to treatments, as well as the closely related question of what kinds of individuals are qualified to provide treatment. This means that if you are working in health promotion, prevention, or intervention efforts across cultures, you may define a health problem as, say, the flu, and understand it to be caused by a particular virus; while the people with whom you are working may define it

[1] From "The Psychology of Encounters," in *The World and the West*, 1953. Oxford: Oxford University Press.

differently—as, for example, a set of symptoms that are the result of improper social relations (e.g., behavior motivated by jealousy). Remember, human beings are biocultural. For this reason, in talking about ethnomedical systems, some theorists have found it useful to make a distinction between a *disease* (an abnormal biomedical state caused by pathogens or physical anomalies) and an *illness* (a culturally defined state of not being well, with many culturally defined causes including biomedical) (Brown 2009). Diseases and illnesses may or may not refer to the same phenomenon.

We can use a table such as the following one to illustrate ethnomedical systems. First let's try one that is Western or biomedical. In the first column, there is a brief list of things that can go wrong or unwell states. In the middle column, these problems are linked to causes, and in the third column, these are in turn linked to treatments.

Now let's look at a hypothetical system that is not primarily Western/biomedical in character. Again, in the first column is a brief list of unwell states, followed by causal and treatment columns.

Functionally, you can see that both systems have the same kinds of elements, and in both cases there is a linkage between the elements. They go together. Perhaps you are looking at these two tables and thinking, "But they aren't the same! One is medicine and the other is . . . myth, or folklore or something." Look again. The first biomedical example and the second are both ethnomedical systems as we have defined the term. The differences have to do with the specific content, and the means by which cause is determined (with respect to cause—in the biomedical case, that includes both research and clinical diagnosis). Where a biomedical system catego-

TABLE 3-2 Hypothetical Nonbiomedical/Ethnomedical System

Problem	Cause	Treatment
Fatigue and body ache	Loss of soul	Spirit healer to intervene and retrieve soul
Seizures	Retaliation by ancestors not properly honored	Ritual (supervised by shaman) to placate and honor ancestors
Stomach pain and vomiting	Imbalance of hot and cold foods and behaviors	Restorative herbal teas for balance, counseling to restore behavioral balance

rizes unwell states based on physical symptoms linked to biological causes, the nonbiomedical system may base its classification on combinations of emotional and physical manifestations, linking these, for example, to spiritual causes, disruptions in harmony, imbalance in a person's lifestyle, or an improper mix of substances and forces. One type of system is based on conclusions from biomedical research using the scientific method developed over time in the Western scientific tradition; the other type is based on conclusions handed down over generations and derived from experience in the world. Both system types, as we will see, combine empirical data and belief in varying proportions.

George Foster, an anthropologist and important figure in the conceptualization of ethnomedical systems (Foster 1976; see also Kleinmann 1980, Foster & Anderson 1978; Murdock 1980; Good 1987; and Rivers 1924), developed a general classification scheme for types of non-Western ethnomedical systems. Foster suggested two general types of non-Western systems: *personalistic* and *naturalistic*.

Personalistic Systems. In a personalistic system, disease is due to the "active, purposeful intervention of an agent" (Foster 1976: 775) where the ill person is the object of action by a sorcerer, spirit, or supernatural force. In keeping with such causal agents, the general pattern of treatment is to block or counter the spiritual or super-

TABLE 3-1 Biomedical/Ethnomedical System

Problem	Cause	Treatment
Flu	Virus	Medication to control fever, rest
Meningitis	Bacteria	Antibacterial medication (antibiotic) to attack invading pathogens
Sickle-cell anemia	Genetic	Genetic testing to assess risk, medication to control disease side effects

natural agent with spiritual or supernatural forces in support of the patient. The center of action, in terms of cause and treatment, is not necessarily within the patient, but in the supernatural world.[2] According to Foster's typology, personalistic ethnomedical systems are also *comprehensive* in the sense that they are a subset of the general system of causality for all things as constructed by those cultures. This portrayal of totalizing or comprehensive witchcraft systems, however, has since been criticized by many scholars for overemphasizing the element of witchcraft as opposed to other aspects of these ethnomedical systems that do not involve witchcraft (see, for example, Pool 1994; Yoder 1982, 1981). In any case, ethnomedical systems that incorporate witchcraft or sorcery include the Azande of Sudan whose traditional belief system, described in detail by Evans-Pritchard (1937) involved the presence of witchcraft and the practice of consulting oracles to identify the source of the witchcraft when a person experienced misfortune or harm, including illness. Other African ethnomedical systems include elements of witchcraft and sorcery as well, which has been a factor, for example, in the popular understanding of HIV/AIDS in Zimbabwe as well as other countries (see Rodlach 2007).

Naturalistic Systems. In a naturalistic system, by contrast, disease is explained by the impersonal actions of systems—usually, says Foster, based on old historical systems of great civilizations, such as the balance of yin and yang in Chinese philosophy (see Box 3-1), or generalized systems of hot/cold balance. Illnesses arise when people are out of balance physically, spiritually, or in some other way. Thus the pattern of treatment is to restore balance through various combinations of herbal medicinals, meditation, diet, lifestyle changes, or other actions. While Foster calls naturalistic systems "restricted" in contrast to personalistic systems, in the sense that causality is specific to the health conditions, that is actually not clear. Some balance-related cultural systems are certainly total cultural systems, not just related to health—this would include the Chinese system, for example.

---

[2] Much of this basic description of African systems, in particular, was influenced by the seminal work of anthropologist E.E. Evans-Pritchard (1937).

BOX 3-1 The Chinese System of Yin-Yang

During the Han dynasty in China (207 BCE–9 ACE), philosophers attempted to integrate many competing explanations regarding the nature of the universe and the cause of worldly phenomena and change. Two basic constructs arose from that effort. The first was the principle of *yin-yang*, opposing forces in the universe that complement each other, where:

- Yin = the female force, the moon, cold, darkness, material form, and other similar aspects.
- Yang = the male force, the sun, creation, heat, light, and similar aspects.

Note that Chinese cultural gender roles are very evident in these principles.

The second was the principle of *wu-hsing*, the five material agents through which the forces of yin and yang operate in the world. These five material agents are wood, fire, earth, metal, and water, and there is an order of relations between them:

Wood gives rise to fire, fire gives rise to earth, earth gives rise to metal, metal gives rise to water, water gives rise to earth, etc.) or the order by which they are conquered by one another: fire is conquered by water, water is conquered by earth, earth is conquered by wood, wood is conquered by metal, and metal is conquered by fire, etc. Each of these orders can be used to explain the progression of change in just about everything.

Sources: The World Civilizations Internet Classroom at Washington State University, www.wsu.edu:8080/~dee/CHPHIL/WUHSING .HTM, and www.wsu.edu:8080/~dee/CHPHIL/YINYANG .HTM.

In addition, personalistic systems as defined by Foster would seem to differ from what could be called "supernatural" or "spiritist" systems, which involve supernatural forces that may be called into play for purposes of healing, but do not involve intentional infliction of harm by one person to another via the use of supernatural forces as implied in a personalistic system. Spiritist systems could include the Latin American/Caribbean examples of Candomblé and Santeria—both of which are strongly influenced by African religious systems (e.g.,

FIGURE 3-1 Restoring Balance (India)

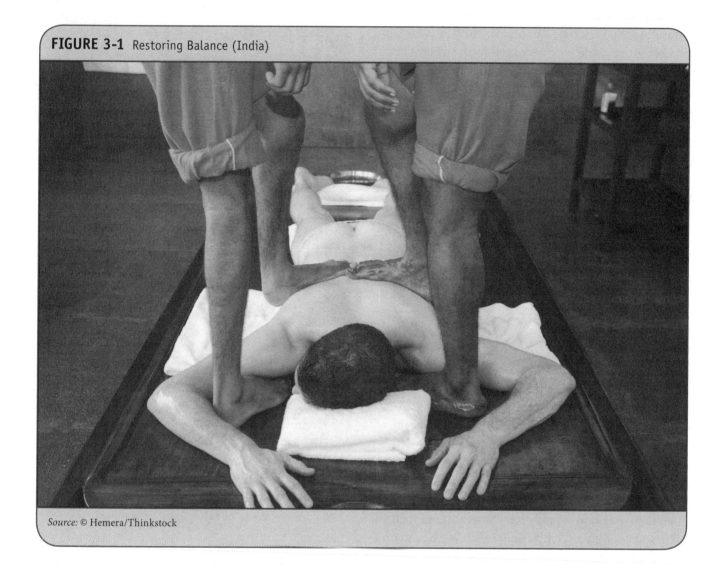

Source: © Hemera/Thinkstock

Yoruba, Bantu). In Candomblé (primarily found in Brazil), there is one all-powerful god called "Olodumare"; however, there are many lesser spirits called "*orixas*" who are the link between humans and the spirit world. Individuals have personal *orixas*, who are protectors who can be called on to intercede and provide help from the spirit world.

A *very important principle to remember*, however, is that Foster's or any other typology of health belief systems is just an abstraction. A given social or cultural group will rarely operate in reference to a single ethnomedical system. The *norm* for most peoples, Western and non-Western, is multiple and coexisting ethnomedical systems, or some blending of elements from various

types of systems. One system may be dominant, but aspects of other systems are also likely to be included.

The Placebo Effect and Role of Belief—In Any Ethnomedical System. If you think, for example, that some of the non-Western systems you may encounter in this text or others are exotic, be reminded that both American and European cultures were and are full of beliefs and practices that involve the supernatural, or belief in the magical properties of objects and actions. This is what leads to the widely reported placebo effect—the tendency for treatments and pills that have no biochemical or biomedical effect to cause improvement in patient health symptoms anyway. This occurs because of the belief that the treatment or pill has curative properties (because, for example, things that look like pills are supposed to be cures or remedies), or because of the ritual process of going to a doctor itself.[3] There's not much difference between that and the healing dowel given to Laura in the scenario introducing this book. And the placebo effect is very much tied to belief in an ethnomedical system—in the case of pills, the allopathic or biomedical system. Studies have also looked at the impact on treatment of the symbolic presentation of physicians, and the way in which multiple aspects of that presentation (manner, equipment, etc.) create an impression of certainty (see Moerman 2010, 2002) that is communicated to the patient and appears to have a significant effect on healing. The white coat itself is a kind of symbol that, in biomedicine, is part of this presentation.

ETHNOMEDICAL SYSTEMS: NON-WESTERN EXAMPLES

Let's take a look now at a range of health knowledge systems across non-Western cultures.[4]

Ayurvedic Medicine (India)

Ayurveda means knowledge or science of life (NIH/NCCAM; University of Maryland Medical Center). It originates with ancient Vedic culture in India and focuses on prevention and a holistic concept of health accomplished though the maintenance of balance in many areas of life, including thought, diet, lifestyle, and the use of herbs (see Lad 1996/2003). Each person has a particular combination of physical, mental, and emotional characteristics, which, together, form that person's constitution or energy pattern. Diagnosis within Ayruvedic medicine involves finding out the imbalance(s) leading to disease. Two ancient books, dating from around 600 BCE, the *Charka Samhita* and *Susruta Samhita*, are said to be key sources for documenting and outlining Ayurvedic theory and practice.

In the Ayurveda system, the body is comprised of three primary energy types, termed "*dosha*." The three *dosha* are called "Vata," "Pitta," and "Kapha." Each *dosha* represents characteristics derived from the five elements of space, air, fire, water, and earth. Vata is the "subtle energy associated with movement" (Lad 1996/2003: 1), composed of space and air. Pitta is connected to the body's metabolic system, made up of fire and water. Kapha is the energy associated with body structure and is composed of earth and water. Each individual has a specific balance of these forces, and equilibrium between the *dosha* means a healthy state; imbalance leads to disease. Ayurvedic healing therefore means a process of identifying imbalance between the *dosha* and prescribing various therapies, including herbal, to restore the balance.

Treatment differs from Western biomedical (allopathic) medicine in that it does not focus on symptoms and the elimination of pathogens or diseased tissue. Instead, it is an attempt to restore balance in order to strengthen the body's natural healing capability. Treatments may include cleansing, diet and lifestyle changes, and medicinal herbs. In addition, Ayurvedic medicine is often used as a complement to Western biomedicine.

Cambodian/*Khmer* Health Belief Systems

While many Cambodians have been exposed to and use Western biomedicine, the use of both Western and traditional systems would not be uncommon. The traditional system shares some aspects in common with Chinese and other Asian systems in the emphasis on balance—a naturalistic system in Foster's classification. Illness may be attributed to imbalance in natural forces, i.e., a humoral theory of causation (see Kemp & Rasbridge 1999–2004). This is often symbolized or expressed as the influence of wind or *kchall* on blood circulation and thus on illness. Body conditions may also be conceptualized as cold or hot, not necessarily referring to temperatures, but to body states leading to or caused by illness or other changes such as childbirth.

Healing practices may be carried out by family members and by traditional healers or *kruu Khmer*. Some *kruu Khmer* specialize in medicinal practice with a spiritual

---

[3] Although there have been some questions about the findings, a 2010 study showed that placebos were effective in treating irritable bowel syndrome, even when patients knew they were placebos (Kaptchuk et al. 2010).

[4] See www.ethnomed.org/culture.

component, while others specialize in magic with a medicinal component. Healing is typically accompanied by prayer and other spiritual activities. The following are examples (Kemp & Rasbridge 1999–2004):

- *Koo'* (rub) *kchall* (wind) is used to treat a variety of ailments, including fever, upper respiratory infection, nausea, weak heart, and malaise. A coin is dipped in a mentholated medicine and rubbed in one direction (away from the center of the body) in a symmetric pattern on the patient's chest, back, and/or extremities. This is referred to in Western literature as "coining" or "dermabrasion."
- *Jup* (pinch) *kchall* is used to treat headache and malaise. *Jup* includes (1) pinching and thus bruising the bridge of the nose, neck, or chest or (2) the practice of cupping or placing a small candle on the forehead, lighting the candle, and placing a small jar over the candle. The flame consumes the oxygen and creates a vacuum, thus causing a circular contusion.
- *Oyt pleung* (known as moxibustion in the literature) is used to treat gastrointestinal and other disorders. *Oyt pleung* is seldom done in the United States, but the abdomens of many adults will have four to six 1–2-cm round scars resulting from the procedure.
- Massage or manipulation is practiced by *kruu Khmer* and others.
- Traditional or natural medicines are available in stores and from individuals. Such medicines include a wide variety of plant (leaves, bark, extracts) and other substances used singly or in combination. They may be used topically or consumed orally.

Spiritual and specifically medicinal elements are combined in healing practices. As in many Southeast Asian cultures, Buddhism and older animist practices are combined in a syncretic, almost seamless way: for example, amulets, strings, and Buddha images are commonly part of treatment or prevention of illness. Other spiritual and supernatural treatments include blowing on the sick person's body in a prescribed manner and showering or rubbing with spiritually endowed water.

South African Health Belief Systems

Despite the fact that much literature on African ethnomedical systems has focused on the centrality of sorcery and personalistic practices (see, for example, Green 1998; Hammond-Tooke 1989; Caldwell & Caldwell 1993), some anthropologists and researchers argue that a more subtle and layered system of belief and practice is in fact operative. Edward Green (1998), for example, argues for a framework called "indigenous contagion theory." According to Green, indigenous contagion theory includes at least three types of naturalistic and impersonal explanations for disease: (1) naturalistic infection (an indigenous germ theory); (2) mystical contagion or pollution; and (3) environmental dangers—causation via external environmental elements, including air. While many diseases are understood through an indigenous contagion theory perspective, when treatment related to these explanations is not successful, more serious and personalistic causes may be thought to be at work, which would require a whole different set of remedies.

Among the Shona (Zimbabwe and southern Mozambique) and other peoples, one aspect of a naturalistic system is understood to be related to the presence of a *nyoka* or snake in the body, which acts as a kind of bodily guardian (Green, Jurg & Djedje 1994). The *nyoka* has a kind of personality that reacts badly to impurities or pollution of the body. For example, a *nyoka* may contract and cause cramps if bad food or medicine enters the body. Or, *nyoka* may cleanse the body through diarrhea, which is seen as a natural function similar to menstruation for eliminating impurities. In fact, *nyoka* are said to be responsible for menstruation as well, and they twist and turn in pain (from impurities), causing cramps. In general, movement of the *nyoka* is related to many diseases, including diarrhea, stomach ailments, sexually transmitted infections, epilepsy, mental retardation, and others. Green (1996) interprets the *nyoka* as a symbol for an ethnomedical system that places importance on purity and pollution (something like contagion), and on the maintenance of balance—so, it is a naturalistic system.

The snake may even be a figure of speech, a metaphor, used to represent the belief system.

Health Belief Systems in Latin America and the Caribbean

Three major and related health-related ethnomedical systems in Latin America and the Caribbean region have been categorized as *Espiritismo*, *Santería*, and *Curanderismo* (see Trusty, Looby & Singh 2002). Brief descriptions of each are:

- *Espiritismo:* Common in Cuba and Puerto Rico, it is a synthesis of Afro-Caribbean, French, and possibly U.S. spiritualist (from the 19th century) traditions. Key to the belief system is that there is both a supreme being and a world of spirits with influence on health that can be accessed through a medium, typically in a group séance-like setting. The medium becomes possessed by the spirit causing the illness and then talks to the spirit about what it has done to the victim. The spirit then asks for forgiveness. The medium also prescribes herbs, baths, and protective fetishes for the client. Audience participation is important. Espiritismo is a blend of personalistic and naturalistic systems.

- *Santerismo/Santería:* Also found in Cuba and Puerto Rico, it is a blend of West African (especially the Yoruba from Nigeria) and Catholic traditions. It is based on the idea that there are many spirits called "orishas" who are connected to the supreme being and who can be appealed to for help in various dimensions of life. A patient goes through a diagnostic process—often where the diviner/healer casts shells on a mat and looks for the pattern. The process of divination is intended to help reveal the orishas involved in the particular health problem who will then provide a diagnosis and a solution. Sacrifices and gifts are made to honor the orishas as a part of the process. The diviner/healer can also prescribe remedies to prevent future problems, such as herbs or amulets. It is a blend of personalistic and naturalistic systems.

- *Curanderismo:* Found in many parts of Central/Latin America. A healer or *curandero* makes a diagnosis using tarot-type cards, or by sweeping a broken egg or other object across the body of the patient. The idea is that there is a supreme or higher power that is the source of energy, and the *curandero* is simply the instrument of that higher power and is a person trained to restore balance to the patient. The healer intercedes in the world of the divine, accessing the energy to restore health—using chants, prayers, imagery, and specific cures. The healer also focuses on restoring balance in the patient's social and family relations. This is a naturalistic system.

ETHNOMEDICAL SYSTEMS: WESTERN EXAMPLES

Biomedicine

The dominant Western ethnomedical system is biomedicine, a system of knowledge and practice dating back at least to Hippocrates in ancient Greece, and a system built on and integrated closely with science. Perhaps the best way to look at Western, biomedical classifications of disease are to examine key diagnostic texts, such as the International Statistical Classification of Diseases and Related Health Problems and the Diagnostic and Statistical Manual used for mental health conditions (see next chapter). The International Statistical Classification of Diseases (or ICD) is typically followed by the version number, such as ICD-10 for the most recent version. It is developed by the World Health Organization and contains codes for each condition within each of the chapters shown in Table 3-3 so that there is a standardized method for referring to diseases that are diagnosed. The code categories are grouped by symptom and causal clusters.

In short, the biomedical system is primarily based on a classification system tied to biological phenomena—the action of pathogens (viruses, bacteria), cellular or other biomechanical malfunctions, injuries/system damage, and others. Treatment is, of course, directly connected to generalists or specialists trained to address specific kinds of biomedical phenomena.

TABLE 3-3 World Health Organization International Statistical Classification of Diseases-10, General Classifications (Chapters)

Chapter	Blocks	Title
I	A00-B99	Certain infectious and parasitic diseases
II	C00-D48	Neoplasms
III	D50-D89	Diseases of the blood and blood-forming organs and certain disorders involving the immune mechanism
IV	E00-E90	Endocrine, nutritional, and metabolic diseases
V	F00-F99	Mental and behavioral disorders
VI	G00-G99	Diseases of the nervous system
VII	H00-H59	Diseases of the eye and adnexa
VIII	H60-H95	Diseases of the ear and mastoid process
IX	I00-I99	Diseases of the circulatory system
X	J00-J99	Diseases of the respiratory system
XI	K00-K93	Diseases of the digestive system
XII	L00-L99	Diseases of the skin and subcutaneous tissue
XIII	M00-M99	Diseases of the musculoskeletal system and connective tissue
XIV	N00-N99	Diseases of the genitourinary system
XV	O00-O99	Pregnancy, childbirth and the puerperium
XVI	P00-P96	Certain conditions originating in the perinatal period
XVII	Q00-Q99	Congenital malformations, deformations, and chromosomal abnormalities
XVIII	R00-R99	Symptoms, signs, and abnormal clinical and laboratory findings, not elsewhere classified
XIX	S00-T98	Injury, poisoning, and certain other consequences of external causes
XX	V01-Y98	External causes of morbidity and mortality
XXI	Z00-Z99	Factors influencing health status and contact with health services
XXII	U00-U99	Codes for special purposes

Source: World Health Organization © Copyright WHO/DIMDI 1994/2006

CHICKEN OR EGG? ETHNOMEDICAL SYSTEMS AND THE GENERATION OF ILLNESS

Here is a question to consider. Given the role of culture as an interpretive framework that contributes to the way in which people understand their situations, feel about them, and act on them, is an ethnomedical system a *reflection* of beliefs and practices that have developed over time, or can it also *generate* beliefs and practices? Suppose a woman named Samantha is part of a culture that believes there is an illness called "*kwaba*," characterized by emotional flatness, erratic behavior, and stomach pains. *Kwaba* is understood to be the result of ancestors exacting revenge when a family member or family does not pay sufficient attention to them, or when someone just ignores his/her family. If left untreated, it can turn into a full-blown case of *kwaba-mora*, with hallucinations, convulsions, and body pain. Now suppose Samantha has just left a very bad, abusive relationship where, in fact, she didn't spend all that much time with her family because of the demands of her partner. After the trauma of leaving the relationship, she does feel emotionally flat. Maybe some days she wants to go out and act wild, and other days she just wants to closet herself in her apartment. She begins to think about her symptoms, and they fit what she understands to be an illness or a syndrome that has a name and a diagnosis in her culture. Then she begins, in her mind, to attach other symptoms to this pattern. She notices, for example, pain in her stomach. She now begins to act like she is ill (see Chapter 5 for a discussion of the sick role), and rushes to find a *thallo*, a kind of healer in her culture that specializes in illnesses resulting from problems with ancestors and family. For all intents and purposes, she has *kwaba*.

What is interesting here is the role the ethnomedical category *kwaba* has played in the way she organizes the symptoms she feels, to the point that she is experiencing *kwaba* the way it is described. If there were no illness called *kwaba* in her culture, she may very well not have linked her symptoms together nor felt like something was wrong. Not only that, but organizing her symptoms that way makes sense, because it fits within larger cultural systems of belief.

Public health anthropologist Robert Hahn (1997) has called this the "nocebo effect" (in contrast to the placebo effect), where expectations generated via an ethnomedical system create negative outcomes. In other words, if a cultural knowledge system provides a label and a descriptive category, this may prompt the category to be filled in by people's experience because it allows people to organize their experience into something meaningful. It doesn't invalidate peoples' experiences at all; it just groups them, so that the categorization of experience becomes what sociologist Emile Durkheim called a "social fact." Some of the conditions discussed in Chapter 4 under "Culture-Bound or Culture-Specific Syndromes" fall into this category.

CASE STUDY:

A Classic Example of the Clash of Ethnomedical Systems: Lia Lee, a Hmong Child with Epilepsy

Perhaps one of the most profoundly documented cases of a clash between two ethnomedical systems and the social and health consequences of that clash concerns the story of a young Hmong immigrant girl in California who had epilepsy. This tragic but revealing story is recounted by Anne Fadiman in *The Spirit Catches You and You Fall Down: A Hmong Child, Her American Doctors, and the Collision of Two Cultures* (Fadiman 1997).

The Hmong—Background. Before proceeding any further, you may be wondering: Who are the Hmong? They are a Southeast Asian population that originated in China and eventually lived in the mountainous regions of Laos, Thailand, and Vietnam. Historically, the Hmong lived in small villages of about 20 households, in high and remote mountain areas. Hmong society was patriarchal, clan based, with multiple generations and family members living in the same household. Villages subsisted on small-scale agriculture. The Hmong language is Sino-Tibetan, but there was no written language until a Romanized alphabet was developed by missionaries in the 1950s.

With respect to religion and its relationship to the ethnomedical system, many Hmong in the United States have become Christian. However, the Hmong who first came to the United States were largely animist and traditionally practiced ancestor worship. Hmong people believed in multiple spirits present in everyday life, and in the existence of supernatural power. Very importantly, the Hmong believe in the existence of multiple souls within each individual, a belief that plays an important role in the etiology of disease and in healing. Shamans (indigenous healers—see Chapter 6) are central to healing, in large part because they are viewed as capable of traveling in the world of spirits. In the beyond or supernatural world live the souls of the dead and the souls of those waiting to be born. Three days after birth, a Hmong baby is given a soul-calling ceremony, in which the baby is first given a name. A necklace is placed around the baby's neck to keep the soul (called a "*plig*").

When someone is sick, a shaman is called to perform a soul-calling ceremony. A shaman goes into trance reinstate a wandering soul, which is possible cause of the illness. Another ceremony or healing practice involves magic to pull the bad spirit from the body of a sick person. Herbal medicines are also used.

Migration to the United States. The Hmong population came to the United States as refugees, a direct consequence of the Vietnam War. During the war, the United States trained a secret Hmong army to disrupt supply lines coming down the Ho Chi Minh trail from North Vietnam, which passed through remote mountainous areas in Laos. The Hmong army was widely known for its courage in fighting much better equipped Vietnamese soldiers, and they also rescued numerous downed U.S. pilots who had flown bombing sorties in Laos targeting the supply trail. When the Communists took over in Vietnam, then Laos in 1975, both governments persecuted the Hmong, and many tried to flee across the borders to refugee camps in Thailand. Since 1976, many Hmong from these camps have been resettled in the United States, most notably in central California, Minnesota, and Wisconsin, though there were resettled Hmong in San Diego, California, Providence, Rhode Island, and other locations as well. When they arrived, most Hmong had little experience with Western culture, including the biomedical system. Life in the United States was difficult at first. Many Hmong were not literate; elders did not learn English, and had few job skills.

(Continues)

The pattern of extended family living and clan social structure was harder to practice in the United States. Many Hmong were exposed to formal education for the first time. Eventually, adaptations were made, and Hmong children attended and often did well in school. In 2002, the first Hmong state senator was elected in Minnesota. The Hmong New Year and other festivals remain important wherever the Hmong are.

The Story. Fadiman's *The Spirit Catches You and You Fall Down*, is a story of a clash between one ethnomedical system—that of the refugee Hmong community—and the biomedical framework under which the doctors and hospital operated. The clash came over a little child with epilepsy, viewed one way by the Hmong and another by the medical system. A young Hmong girl named Lia Lee was diagnosed with severe epilepsy by a hospital in Fresno, California. In the Hmong ethnomedical system, however, epileptic symptoms meant something very different than the biomedical understanding of epilepsy. First, according to Hmong belief, epileptic symptoms were viewed as the result of soul loss, where a soul must have been frightened out of Lia's body by a sudden or dramatic situation. Epilepsy was known to the Hmong as *qaub dab peg*, or, in English, a spirit catches you and you fall down. The sudden event identified by the Lee family was a loud door slam, which caused her soul to flee and precipitated her seizures. Second, epileptic seizures were also viewed by the Hmong as a kind of blessing, as evidence that the person can perceive things other people cannot, and therefore has a special, spiritual capability. To cure the seizures and return Lia's soul to her, a shaman (called a "*txiv neeb*") was needed to perform a soul calling.

The difference between the treatment prescribed by doctors at the hospital and the treatment prescribed under the Hmong system was dramatic—though the Lee family did believe that something needed to be done to address the increasingly severe seizures. There was misunderstanding, miscommunication, and frustration on both sides. The Lee family did not always understand the changing regimen of medications for their daughter, and they believed that some of the medications were in fact causing harm—a belief that had some basis, since Lia suffered from side effects including, eventually, an infection that caused a coma and eventual vegetative state. The doctors did not understand the Hmong ethnomedical beliefs about epilepsy and viewed the Lee family as resistant, even to the point that Lia was taken from her family for a period of time by social services.

At the time, few resources were available to bridge the gap in understanding. Even though both the biomedical doctors and the Lee family came to some understanding of each other's treatment approach and reasons, this did not really occur until the story reached its tragic conclusion. It is a case in point for the need to understand the diversity in health beliefs and practices, and to take a collaborative approach to treatment that recognizes the legitimacy of different systems.

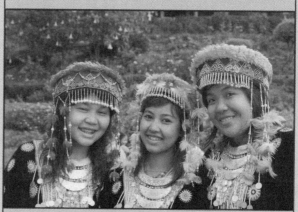

FIGURE 3-2 Hmong Girls at New Year Festival in Laos

Source: © Artur Bogacki/ShutterStock, Inc

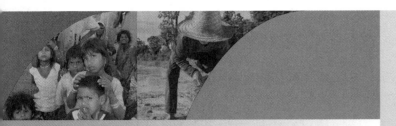

QUESTIONS

1. Do you or anyone you know use an alternative treatment for any health condition? If so, what is it based on? (What is the underlying ethnomedical system?)

2. What are some examples of the nocebo effect that you have seen or heard about?

3. If you watch late-night television, you have undoubtedly seen the proliferation of pharmaceutical advertisements and the issues they claim to treat. What effect do you think these have on diagnosis and treatment?

4. Can you call biomedicine an ethnomedical system? Why or why not?

5. What are some of the similarities and differences in the non-Western ethnomedical systems profiled briefly in this chapter?

REFERENCES

Brown, P., ed. 2009. *Understanding and Applying Medical Anthropology*, 2nd ed. New York: McGraw-Hill.

Caldwell, J.C. and P. Caldwell. 1993. "The Nature and Limits of the Sub-Saharan African AIDS Epidemic: Evidence from Geographic and Other Patterns." *Population and Development Review* 19(4): 817–848.

Evans-Pritchard, E.E. 1937. *Witchcraft, Oracles and Magic among the Azande*. Oxford, England: Clarendon Press.

Fadiman, A. 1997. *The Spirit Catches You and You Fall Down: A Hmong Child, Her American Doctors, and the Collision of Two Cultures*. New York: Farrar, Straus and Giroux.

Foster, G.M. 1976. "Disease Etiologies in Non-Western Medical Systems." *American Anthropologist* 78: 773–782.

Foster, G.M., and B.G. Anderson. 1978. *Medical Anthropology*. New York: John Wiley & Sons.

Good, C. 1987. *Ethnomedical Systems in Africa: Patterns of Traditional Medicine in Rural and Urban Kenya*. New York: Guilford Press.

Green, E. 1996. "Purity, Pollution and the Invisible Snake in Southern Africa." *Medical Anthropology* 17 (1): 83–100.

Green, E.C. 1998. "Etiology in Human and Animal Ethnomedicine." *Agriculture and Human Values* 15: 127–131.

Green, E.C., A. Jurg, and A. Djedje. (1994). "The Snake in the Stomach: Child Diarrhea in Central Mozambique." *Medical Anthropology Quarterly* 8 (1): 4–24.

Hahn, R. 1997. "The Nocebo Phenomenon: Concept, Evidence and Implications for Public Health." *Preventive Medicine* 26 (5) 607–611.

Hammond-Tooke, W.D. 1989. *Rituals and Medicines*. Johannesburg, South Africa: A.D. Donker.

Kaptchuk, T.J., E. Friedlander, J.M. Kelley, N.M. Sanchez, E. Kokkotou, J.P. Singer, M. Kowalczykowski, F.G. Miller, I. Kirsch, and A.J. Lembo. 2010. "Placebos without Deception: A Randomized Control Trial in Irritable Bowel Syndrome." *PloS One* 5 (12): e15591. doi:10.1371/journal.pone.0015591

Kemp, C., and L. Rasbridge. 1999–2004. *Asian Health Resources for Cross-Cultural Care and Prevention*. Baylor University, accessed February–March 2010, http://bearspace.baylor.edu/Charles_Kemp/www/asian_health.html.

Kleinman, A. 1980. *Patients and Healers in the Context of Culture: An Exploration of the Borderland between Anthropology, Medicine, and Psychiatry*. Berkeley: University of California Press.

Lad, V. 1996/2003. *Ayurveda: A Brief Introduction and Guide*. Albuquerque, NM: The Ayurvedic Press.

Moerman, D. 2002. *Meaning, Medicine, and the Placebo Effect*. Cambridge: Cambridge University Press.

Moerman, D. 2010. "Doctors and Patients: The Role of Clinicians in the Placebo Effect." In *Understanding and Applying Medical Anthropology*, 2nd ed., edited by P.J. Brown and R. Barrett. Boston: McGraw-Hill, pages 133–140.

Murdock, G.P. 1980. *Theories of Illness: A World Survey*. Pittsburgh: University of Pittsburgh Press.

National Institutes of Health/National Center for Complementary and Alternative Medicine, accessed March 2010, www.nccam.nih.gov/health/ayurveda

Pool, R. 1994. "On the Creation and Dissolution of Ethnomedical Systems in the Medical Ethnography of Africa." *Africa: Journal of the International African Institute* 64 (1): 1–20.

Rivers, W.H.R. 1924. *Medicine, Magic and Religion*. London: Kegan Paul.

Rodlach, A. 2007. *Witches, Westerners and HIV: AIDS and Cultures of Blame in Africa*. Walnut Creek, CA: Left Coast Press.

Trusty, J., E. Looby, and D. Singh. 2002. *Multicultural Counseling: Context, Theory and Practice, and Competence*. Huntington, NY: Nova Science Publishers, Inc.

University of Maryland Medical Center Alternative Medicine site, accessed March 2010, www.umm.edu/altmed/articles/ayurveda-000348.htm.

Yoder, P.S. 1981. "Knowledge of Illness and Medicine among Cokwe of Zaire." *Social Science and Medicine (special issue)* 15B: 237–245.

Yoder, P.S. 1982. "Introduction." In *African Health and Healing Systems: Proceedings of a Symposium*, edited by P.S. Yoder, 1–20. Los Angeles: Crossroads Press.

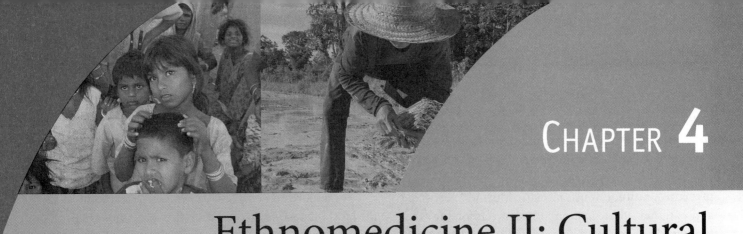

CHAPTER 4

Ethnomedicine II: Cultural Systems of Psychology and Mental/Emotional Health

"All the lessons of psychiatry, psychology, social work, indeed culture, have taught us over the last hundred years that it is the acceptance of differences, not the search for similarities which enables people to relate to each other in their personal or family lives."

—John Ralston Saul, *Reflection of a Siamese Twin*

Now we can extend the discussion of ethnomedical systems in Chapter 3 to the way in which such systems, across cultures, address conditions that are commonly viewed as psychological or emotional from a Western perspective. The division is an arbitrary one, because many ethnomedical systems do not include any such distinction, and the boundaries have been blurred even within the biomedical paradigm. Nevertheless, these kinds of conditions have been categorized together and examined within subdisciplines such as ethnopsychiatry, cross-cultural psychology, and transcultural psychiatry. If we start with the well-vs.-unwell distinction basic to the idea of an ethnomedical system, the focus here is on unwell states whose primary causes do not originate in the body itself. This would mean—with a reminder that our terminology must be loosely interpreted—conditions identified within a particular culture that differ from a normative mental or emotional state, *whatever that is considered to be.* As you will see, this does not mean that

a given psychological or emotional condition is not also experienced through the body as physical symptoms.

THE CULTURAL CONSTRUCTION OF MENTAL/EMOTIONAL ILLNESS

Like physically centered illnesses, *ethnopsychiatric* conditions may or may not have a biological origin, or they may involve a specific organization (lumping together) of biological and emotional symptoms. Anything defined as an abnormal mental/emotional state is also likely to involve a cultural judgment and therefore may say a lot about cultural values and beliefs as a whole at particular moments in history. For a long time in the United States, for example, women were viewed as naturally prone to hysteria, and as such any expression of that could have been considered normal for women, but not for men. Individuals who at one time may have been viewed as spiritually gifted or clairvoyant, or even as prophets or religious figures, might be viewed in more contemporary times as psychotic—as seeing visions.

Here is a favorite example: In 1851, a Dr. Samuel Cartwright (1851) defined a psychopathic condition that he called "drapetomania," affecting African American slaves. Drapetomania was "the disease causing negroes to run away" (Ibid, 691). Imagine that! Trying to run away from enslavement—as an illness! It was, according to Cartwright, a curable disease of the mind, involving sulkiness and dissatisfaction prior to running away, that could be brought on when white slave owners treated slaves too much like human beings, or on the other hand when they were overly cruel and brutal. The appropriate preventive attitude was a measured form of restricted and paternal subordination aimed at reinforcing what Cartwright viewed as the slaves' divinely ordained submissive state. In the same volume, he coined another condition afflicting slaves called "dysaethesia aethiopica," characterized by a state of half-sleep and a physical or nervous insensibility that caused them to behave like rascals—causing mischief and "breaking, wasting and destroying everything they handle," even tearing, burning or rending their own clothing, and "slighting their work, cutting up corn, cane or cotton when hoeing it" and generally "raining disturbances." Not to dwell on the obvious, but what do you think lay behind any of these "symptoms"?

For a more contemporary example, perhaps one of the most interesting documents is the voluminous manual used in the United States and Western biomedicine to diagnose mental health conditions. It is the *Diagnostic and Statistical Manual (DSM)* published by the American Psychiatric Association. Like the International Statistical Classification of Diseases (see Chapter 3), the DSM is usually referred to by the version being used. The most common version for many years was the DSM-IV, but this is now being replaced by the DSM V. The DSM

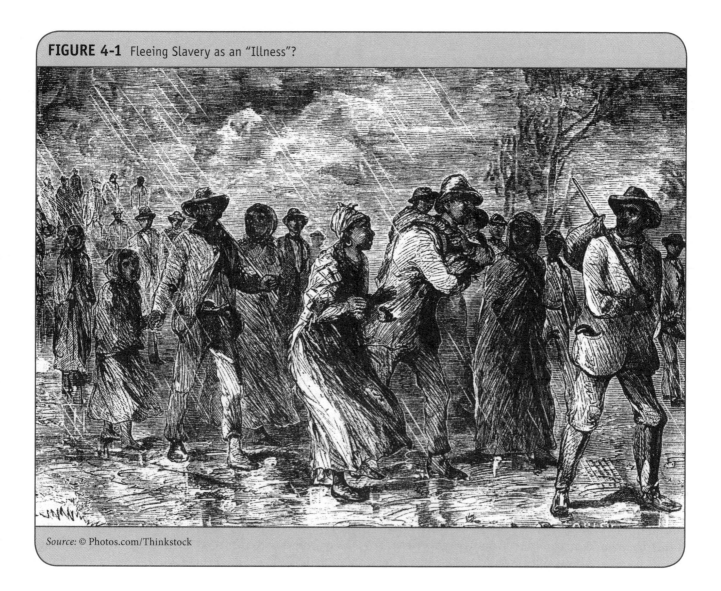

FIGURE 4-1 Fleeing Slavery as an "Illness"?

Source: © Photos.com/Thinkstock

is a reference book for mental health conditions that are viewed in Western/biomedicine as abnormal, with detailed descriptions of the etiology (cause), symptoms, and treatment for each condition—an ethnopsychiatric system-in-a-book, so to speak. While of course it is based on extensive scientific/clinical research and experience, the symptoms and descriptions for many conditions offer a fascinating glimpse of the way in which such conditions can be shaped by cultural expectations and changes in such expectations. Let's just look at a few conditions.

Antisocial Personality Disorder. According to the DSM-IV (APA 2000), antisocial personality disorder is a disorder characterized by a pervasive pattern of disregarding and violating the rights of others. This pattern must include at least three of the following specific signs and symptoms:

- Failure to conform to social norms with respect to lawful behaviors as indicated by repeatedly performing acts that are grounds for arrest
- Deceitfulness, as indicated by repeatedly lying, use of aliases, or conning others for personal profit or pleasure
- Impulsivity, or failure to think or plan ahead
- Irritability and aggressiveness, as indicated by repeated physical fights or assaults
- Reckless disregard for the safety of self or others
- Consistent irresponsibility, as indicated by repeated failure to sustain consistent work behavior or honor financial obligations
- Lack of remorse, as indicated by being indifferent to or rationalizing having hurt, mistreated, or stolen from another

In addition, the individual diagnosed with antisocial personality disorder must be over 18 and have shown a pattern of these symptoms since age 15 or older.

Now, think about these symptoms. On the one hand, if considered out of any specific context, they do seem to outline a kind of personality that could be viewed as troublesome if not criminal. But the picture changes when context and culture are added. Imagine that you are part of a social or cultural subgroup that is marginalized and has an antagonistic relationship with local police. Add to that a dose of racism or cultural superiority that the police and other government officials—

even public healthcare providers—display towards your group. Add to that the difficulty members of your group have in finding employment, and the generally limited expectations many group members have about a viable socioeconomic future. Now look again at the signs and symptoms of antisocial personality disorder:

- Is it possible that a rational individual (from the marginalized group) with no actual disorder would engage in illegal activity, even repeatedly, in order to obtain money?
- Is it possible that a rational individual (from the marginalized group) with no actual disorder would exhibit frustration, hostility, and aggressiveness?
- Is it possible that a rational individual (from the marginalized group) with no actual disorder would not bother doing much planning for a future he or she could not see?

All are possible, and they illustrate both the potential bias such classifications of disorder have (in this case, they are behaviors that might be out of place among groups who are not in marginalized situations), and the potential for such disorders to mask other social phenomena by focusing primarily on the individual as the culprit. This leaves open the question—are these really disorders of the individuals, or are they related to broader social disorders? And do they reflect a cultural bias towards understanding behavior—whether good or bad—as primarily an outcome of individuals?

Attention Deficit/Hyperactivity Disorder. According to the DSM-IV, this disorder is characterized by two sets of symptoms—inattention and hyperactivity-impulsivity. An affected person can have symptoms of either one. The specific description and criteria are as follows:

For *inattention,* six or more of the following symptoms have persisted for at least 6 months to a degree that is maladaptive and inconsistent with developmental level:

- Often fails to give close attention to details or makes careless mistakes in schoolwork, work, or other activities
- Often has difficulty sustaining attention in tasks or play activities
- Often does not seem to listen when spoken to directly

- Often does not follow through on instructions and fails to finish schoolwork, chores, or duties in the workplace (not due to oppositional behavior or failure to understand instructions)
- Often has difficulty organizing tasks and activities
- Often avoids, dislikes, or is reluctant to engage in tasks that require sustained mental effort (such as schoolwork or homework)
- Often loses things necessary for tasks or activities (e.g., toys, school assignments, pencils, books, or tools)
- Is often easily distracted by extraneous stimuli
- Is often forgetful in daily activities

For *hyperactivity-impulsivity*, six or more of the following symptoms have persisted for at least 6 months to a degree that is maladaptive and inconsistent with developmental level:

Hyperactivity

- Often fidgets with hands or feet or squirms in seat
- Often leaves seat in the classroom or in other situations in which remaining seated is expected
- Often runs about or climbs excessively in situations in which it is inappropriate (in adolescents or adults, may be limited to subjective feelings of restlessness)
- Often has difficulty playing or engaging in leisure activities quietly
- Is often on the go or often acts as if driven by a motor
- Often talks excessively

Impulsivity

- Often blurts out answers before questions have been completed
- Often has difficulty awaiting turn
- Often interrupts or intrudes on others (e.g., butts into conversations or games)

In addition, the following are also requirements of the diagnosis:

- Some hyperactive-impulsive or inattentive symptoms that cause impairment were present before age 7 years.
- Some impairment from the symptoms is present in two or more settings (e.g., at school or work and at home).
- There must be clear evidence of clinically significant impairment in social, academic, or occupational functioning.
- The symptoms do not occur exclusively during the course of a pervasive developmental disorder, schizophrenia, or other psychotic disorder and are not better accounted for by another mental disorder (e.g., mood disorder, anxiety disorder, dissociative disorder, or a personality disorder).

This is undoubtedly a condition that can cause difficulties and impairs appropriate functioning and may in some cases be caused by perinatal complications or brain damage (see U.S. DHHS 1999). But there is room for interpretation. Some elements of hyperactivity, for example, are subjective and depend on culturally related standards for appropriate behavior. Consider "often has difficulty playing or engaging in leisure activities quietly," or "is often on the go or often acts as if driven by a motor," or "often talks excessively." How are these really defined? A relatively quiet child in one culture may be a loud and intrusive one in another. De Ramirez and Shapiro (2005) report on a number of studies showing that teacher ratings of children's behavior using these criteria differ significantly by culture, even contradicting actual videotapes of the behavior. One study comparing teacher ratings of Thai vs. non-Thai U.S. students to direct observations of those students showed that Thai students were rated as more pathological (by attention deficit/hyperactivity disorder criteria) than U.S. students, even though observations indicated otherwise (Weisz et al. 1995). The standards and expectations applied to Thai students were simply different (normative Thai student behavior was quieter and more restrained), such that deviations from that standard stood out more than the same behaviors would for the U.S. students. The same kinds of differences have been identified in teacher ratings of Jamaican vs. African American children (Puig et al. 1999).

FIGURE 4-2 Thai Students

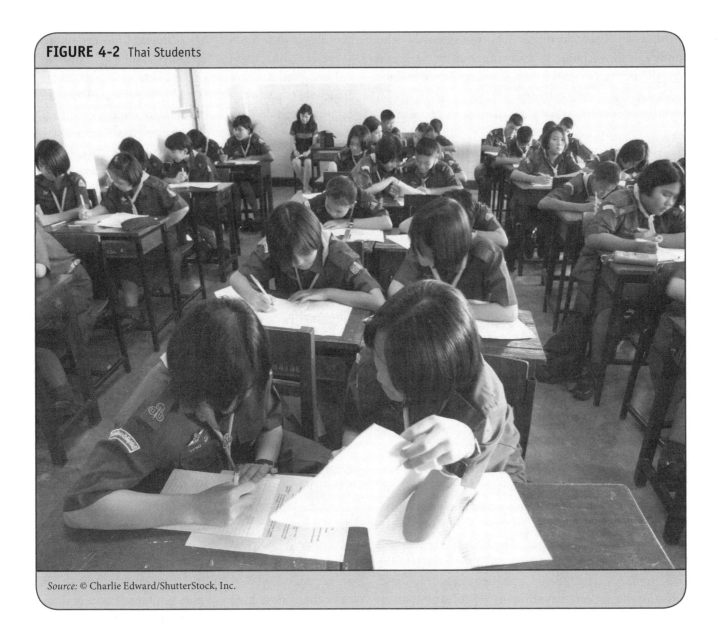

Source: © Charlie Edward/ShutterStock, Inc.

The Question of Universal vs. Culture-Specific Conditions. The existence of culturally constructed mental health conditions leads to a key question: Do all human beings experience the same mental health phenomena, or emotional phenomena? Are these things universal, but perhaps surfacing in different forms? Or are they unique for each culture? The universalist position would argue for the former—that human beings have essentially the same psychological makeup—a position often referred to as "psychic unity." The other position falls more in line with a cultural relativist perspective, in which cultures entail unique patterns of thought and behavior. Or is human experience somewhere in between?

In this book we will take the in-between position, stated as follows: it is not likely that there are completely isolated mental health conditions in just single cultures. Instead, cultures shape how emotions and mental experiences are constructed, named, and given meaning, and the living patterns of specific cultures tend to accentuate particular stressors that may result in mental health issues. There do appear to be some mental health conditions that occur in some form across cultures, and so could be seen as universal conditions. These include depression-like symptoms and schizophrenia. Note that both these conditions have a biochemical and genetic component. Moreover, mental health problems are not exclusive to the developed world. Global measures of the burden of disease demonstrate that emotional and mental health conditions, however defined, occur across cultures and societies (see the World Health Organization Global Burden of Disease at www.who.int/healthinfo/global_burden_disease/en/index.html).

Mental health conditions that appear unique to one or a few cultural groups can be thought of in two ways—as culture-bound syndromes and as conditions that are prompted by specific patterns of social stress and/or ecological contexts. There is clearly an overlap between these two arbitrary categories, but they are useful abstractions to help in understanding. We will take a look at each.

CULTURE-BOUND OR CULTURE-SPECIFIC SYNDROMES

The *McGraw-Hill Dictionary of Scientific and Technical Terms* (Parker 2003) defines a culture-specific syndrome as "any from of disturbed behavior that is specific to a certain cultural system and does not conform to Western classification of diseases" The DSM-IV (American Psychological Association 2000, 844), the first of the DSM volumes to include any specific reference to these, defines culture-bound syndromes as "recurrent, locality-specific patterns of aberrant behavior and troubling experience that may or may not be linked to a particular DSM-IV diagnostic category. Many of these patterns are indigenously considered to be 'illnesses,' or afflictions, and most have local names" (from introductory text, Glossary of Culture Bound Syndromes, DSM-IV, 844). As is evident, both definitions specifically contrast such conditions against Western classifications as listed in the DSM, and in the DSM-IV, these culture-bound syndromes (CBSs) are separated from the main DSM-IV text and shown in Appendix I. The list of culture-bound syndromes is in Box 4-1.

Problems with the Idea of Culture-Bound Syndromes. The DSM-IV use of culture-bound symptoms has been the object of a number of critiques. Charles Hughes (1998), coeditor of one of the important early books on culture-bound symptoms, offers several important critiques: (1) even though the DSM-IV Appendix I includes language about taking cultural factors into account and differing symptoms across cultures, there are no suggested steps for how a provider should incorporate cultural factors into the diagnosis or even learn what those factors are; 2) the cordoning off of culturally influenced symptoms or conditions as by nature specific to certain cultures distorts, in his view, the overlap between some conditions across cultures; and 3) the process of selecting the culture-bound systems in Appendix I is unclear.

If, in this book, we reiterate that all *human beings are cultural*, then it would not make a lot of sense to think of just a few syndromes as culture-bound. The Western biomedical system, as we have noted, is also an ethnomedical system, and by definition rooted in cultural factors. According to Hughes (ibid., 420), "The culture bound syndromes [in the DSM-IV appendix] are important not as a museum of exotic, static, bounded entities, but as illustrations of a generic way of thinking about relationships between psychopathology and cultural context (citing Kirmayer 1990, 1991; Hughes 1994)."

Following the same logic, it may be better to use the term *culture-reactive syndrome* than *culture bound syndrome* (Simons & Hughes 1985; Winkelman 2009), as a better way of acknowledging that such syndromes are a product of a biocultural interaction, and that if more than one culture presents similar stressors or shaping conditions, that the syndrome may occur in all of them—not just one.

MENTAL HEALTH CONDITIONS RESULTING FROM CULTURALLY LINKED SOCIAL STRESSORS AND PRACTICES

Let's assume, then, that most conditions referred to as culture bound (or culture reactive) syndromes are the outcome of unique kinds of social stressors. These could include gender rules and requirements, strict social or family obligation systems, specific patterns of social marginalization and hierarchy, immigration/acculturation trauma, and others.

BOX 4-1 DSM-IV Glossary of Culture-Bound Syndromes from Appendix I: Outline for Cultural Formulation and Glossary of Culture-Bound Syndromes

Amok—A dissociative episode characterized by a period of brooding followed by an outburst of violent, aggressive, or homicidal behavior directed at people and objects. The episode tends to be precipitated by a perceived slight or insult and seems to be prevalent only among males. The episode is often accompanied by persecutory ideas, automatism, amnesia, exhaustion, and a return to premorbid state following the episode. Some instances of amok may occur during a brief psychotic episode or constitute the onset or an exacerbation of a chronic psychotic process. The original reports that used this term were from Malaysia. A similar behavior pattern is found in Laos, Philippines, Polynesia (*cafard* or *cathard*), Papua New Guinea, and Puerto Rico (*mal de pelea*), and among the Navajo (*iich'aa*).

Ataque de nervios—An idiom of distress principally reported among Latinos from the Caribbean but recognized among many Latin American and Latin Mediterranean groups. Commonly reported symptoms include uncontrollable shouting, attacks of crying, trembling, heat in the chest rising into the head, and verbal or physical aggression. Dissociative experiences, seizurelike or fainting episodes, and suicidal gestures are prominent in some attacks but absent in others. A general feature of an *ataque de nervios* is a sense of being out of control. *Ataques de nervios* frequently occur as a direct result of a stressful event relating to the family (e.g., news of the death of a close relative, a separation or divorce from a spouse, conflicts with a spouse or children, or witnessing an accident involving a family member). People may experience amnesia for what occurred during the *ataque de nervios*, but they otherwise return rapidly to their usual level of functioning. Although descriptions of some *ataques de nervios* most closely fit with the DSM-IV description of panic attacks, the association of most *ataques* with a precipitating event and the frequent absence of the hallmark symptoms of acute fear or apprehension distinguish them from panic disorder. *Ataques* span the range from normal expressions of distress not associated with having a mental disorder to symptom presentations associated with the diagnoses of anxiety, mood, dissociative, or somatoform disorders.

Bilis and *colera* (**also referred to as** *muina*)—The underlying cause of these syndromes is thought to be strongly experienced anger or rage. Anger is viewed among many Latino groups as a particularly powerful emotion that can have direct effects on the body and can exacerbate existing symptoms. The major effect of anger is to disturb core body balances (which are understood as a balance between hot and cold in the body and between the material and spiritual aspects of the body). Symptoms can include acute nervous tension, headache, trembling, screaming, stomach disturbances, and, in more severe cases, loss of consciousness. Chronic fatigue may result from the acute episode.

Boufée delirante—A syndrome observed in West Africa and Haiti. This French term refers to a sudden outburst of agitated and aggressive behavior, marked confusion, and psychomotor excitement. It may sometimes be accompanied by visual and auditory hallucinations or paranoid ideation. These episodes may resemble an episode of brief psychotic disorder.

Brain *fag*—A term initially used in West Africa to refer to a condition experienced by high school or university students in response to the challenges of schooling. Symptoms include difficulties in concentrating, remembering, and thinking. Students often state that their brains are fatigued. Additional somatic symptoms are usually centered around the head and neck and include pain, pressure or tightness, blurring of vision, heat, or burning. Brain tiredness or fatigue from too much thinking is an idiom of distress in many cultures, and resulting syndromes can resemble certain anxiety, depressive, and somatoform disorders.

Dhat—A folk diagnostic term used in India to refer to severe anxiety and hypochondriacal concerns associated with the discharge of semen, whitish discoloration of the urine, and feelings of weakness and exhaustion. Similar to *jiryan* (India), *sukra prameha* (Sri Lanka), and *shen-k'uei* (China).

Falling-out or blacking out—These episodes occur primarily in southern United States and Caribbean groups. They are characterized by a sudden collapse, which sometimes occurs without warning but sometimes is preceded by feelings of dizziness or swimming in the head. The individual's eyes are usually open but the person claims an inability to see. The person usually hears and understands what is occurring around him or her but feels powerless to move. This may correspond to a diagnosis of conversion disorder or a dissociative disorder.

Ghost sickness—A preoccupation with death and the deceased (sometimes associated with witchcraft) frequently observed among members of many American Indian tribes. Various symptoms can be attributed to ghost sickness, including bad

(Continues)

BOX 4-1 *(Continued)*

dreams, weakness, feelings of danger, loss of appetite, fainting, dizziness, fear, anxiety, hallucinations, loss of consciousness, confusion, feelings of futility, and a sense of suffocation.

Hwa-byung (also known as *wool-hwa-byung*)—A Korean folk syndrome translated into English as anger syndrome and attributed to the suppression of anger. The symptoms include insomnia, fatigue, panic, fear of impending death, dysphoric affect, indigestion, anorexia, dyspnea, palpitations, generalized aches and pains, and a feeling of a mass in the epigastrium.

Koro—A term, probably of Malaysian origin, that refers to an episode of sudden and intense anxiety that the penis (or, in females, the vulva and nipples) will recede into the body and possibly cause death. The syndrome is reported in south and east Asia, where it is known by a variety of local terms, such as *shuk yang, shook yong,* and *suo yang* (Chinese); *jinjinia bemar* (Assam); or *rok-joo* (Thailand). It is occasionally found in the West. Koro at times occurs in localized epidemic form in east Asian areas. This diagnosis is included in the *Chinese Classification of Mental Disorders*, 2nd ed. (Chinese Association of Psychiatry 1995).

Latah—Hypersensitivity to sudden fright, often with echopraxia, echolalia, command obedience, and dissociative or trancelike behavior. The term *latah* is of Malaysian or Indonesian origin, but the syndrome has been found in many parts of the world. Other terms for this condition are *amurakh, irkunii, ikota, olan, myriachit,* and *menkeiti* (Siberian groups); *bah tschi, bah-tsi,* and *baah-ji* (Thailand); *imu* (Ainu, Sakhalin, Japan); and *mali-mali* and *silok* (Philippines). In Malaysia it is more frequent in middle-aged women.

Locura—A term used by Latinos in the United States and Latin America to refer to a severe form of chronic psychosis. The condition is attributed to an inherited vulnerability, to the effect of multiple life difficulties, or to a combination of both factors. Symptoms exhibited by persons with locura include incoherence, agitation, auditory and visual hallucinations, inability to follow rules of social interaction, unpredictability, and possible violence.

Mal de ojo—A concept widely found in Mediterranean cultures and elsewhere in the world. *Mal de ojo* is a Spanish phrase translated into English as evil eye. Children are especially at risk. Symptoms include fitful sleep, crying without apparent cause, diarrhea, vomiting, and fever in a child or infant. Sometimes adults (especially females) have the condition.

Nervios—A common idiom of distress among Latinos in the United States and Latin America. A number of other ethnic groups have related, though often somewhat distinctive, ideas of nerves (such as *nevra* among Greeks in North America). *Nervios* refers both to a general state of vulnerability to stressful life experiences and to a syndrome brought on by difficult life circumstances. The term *nervios* includes a wide range of symptoms of emotional distress, somatic disturbance, and inability to function. Common symptoms include headaches and brain aches, irritability, stomach disturbances, sleep difficulties, nervousness, easy tearfulness, inability to concentrate, trembling, tingling sensations, and *mareos* (dizziness with occasional vertigo-like exacerbations). *Nervios* tends to be an ongoing problem, although variable in the degree of disability manifested. Nervios is a very broad syndrome that spans the range from cases free of a mental disorder to presentations resembling adjustment, anxiety, depressive, dissociative, somatoform, or psychotic disorders. Differential diagnosis will depend on the constellation of symptoms experienced, the kind of social events that are associated with the onset and progress of *nervios*, and the level of disability experienced.

Pibloktoq—An abrupt dissociative episode accompanied by extreme excitement of up to 30 minutes' duration and frequently followed by convulsive seizures and coma lasting up to 12 hours. This is observed primarily in arctic and subarctic Eskimo communities, although regional variations in name exist. The individual may be withdrawn or mildly irritable for a period of hours or days before the attack and will typically report complete amnesia for the attack. During the attack, the individual may tear off his or her clothing, break furniture, shout obscenities, eat feces, flee from protective shelters, or perform other irrational or dangerous acts.

Qi-gong psychotic reaction—A term describing an acute, time-limited episode characterized by dissociative, paranoid, or other psychotic or nonpsychotic symptoms that may occur after participation in the Chinese folk health-enhancing practice of *qi-gong* (exercise of vital energy). Especially vulnerable are individuals who become overly involved in the practice. This diagnosis is included in the *Chinese Classification of Mental Disorders*, 2nd ed.

Root work—A set of cultural interpretations that ascribe illness to hexing, witchcraft, sorcery, or the evil influence of another person. Symptoms may include generalized anxiety and gastrointestinal complaints (e.g., nausea, vomiting, diarrhea), weakness, dizziness, the fear of being poisoned, and sometimes fear of being killed (voodoo death). Roots, spells, or hexes can be put or placed on other persons, causing a variety of emotional and psychological problems. The hexed person may even

BOX 4-1 (Continued)

fear death until the root has been eliminated, usually through the work of a root doctor (a healer in this tradition), who can also be called on to bewitch an enemy. Root work is found in the southern United States among both African American and European American populations and in Caribbean societies. It is also known as *mal puesto* or *brujeria* in Latino societies.

Sangue dormido (sleeping blood)—This syndrome is found among Portuguese Cape Verde Islanders (and immigrants from there to the United States) and includes pain, numbness, tremor, paralysis, convulsions, stroke, blindness, heart attack, infection, and miscarriage.

Shenjing shuairuo (neurasthenia)—In China, a condition characterized by physical and mental fatigue, dizziness, headaches, other pains, concentration difficulties, sleep disturbance, and memory loss. Other symptoms include gastrointestinal problems, sexual dysfunction, irritability, excitability, and various signs suggesting disturbance of the autonomic nervous system. In many cases, the symptoms would meet the criteria for a DSM-IV mood or anxiety disorder. This diagnosis is included in the *Chinese Classification of Mental Disorders*, 2nd ed.

Shen-k'uei (Taiwan); *shenkui* (China)—A Chinese folk label describing marked anxiety or panic symptoms with accompanying somatic complaints for which no physical cause can be demonstrated. Symptoms include dizziness, backache, fatigability, general weakness, insomnia, frequent dreams, and complaints of sexual dysfunction (such as premature ejaculation and impotence). Symptoms are attributed to excessive semen loss from frequent intercourse, masturbation, nocturnal emission, or passing of white turbid urine believed to contain semen. Excessive semen loss is feared because of the belief that it represents the loss of one's vital essence and can thereby be life threatening.

Shin-byung—A Korean folk label for a syndrome in which initial phases are characterized by anxiety and somatic complaints (general weakness, dizziness, fear, anorexia, insomnia, gastrointestinal problems), with subsequent dissociation and possession by ancestral spirits.

Spell—A trance state in which individuals communicate with deceased relatives or with spirits. At times this state is associated with brief periods of personality change. This culture-specific syndrome is seen among African Americans and European Americans from the southern United States. Spells are not considered to be medical events in the folk tradition but may be misconstrued as psychotic episodes in clinical settings.

Susto (fright or soul loss)—A folk illness prevalent among some Latinos in the United States and among people in Mexico, Central America, and South America. *Susto* is also referred to as *"espanto," "pasmo," "tripa ida," "pérdida del alma,"* and *"chibih." Susto* is an illness attributed to a frightening event that causes the soul to leave the body and results in unhappiness and sickness. Individuals with *susto* also experience significant strains in key social roles. Symptoms may appear any time from days to years after the fright is experienced. It is believed that in extreme cases, *susto* may result in death. Typical symptoms include appetite disturbances, inadequate or excessive sleep, troubled sleep or dreams, feeling of sadness, lack of motivation to do anything, and feelings of low self-worth or dirtiness. Somatic symptoms accompanying *susto* include muscle aches and pains, headache, stomachache, and diarrhea. Ritual healings are focused on calling the soul back to the body and cleansing the person to restore bodily and spiritual balance. Different experiences of *susto* may be related to major depressive disorder, posttraumatic stress disorder, and somatoform disorders. Similar etiological beliefs and symptom configurations are found in many parts of the world.

Taijin kyofusho—A culturally distinctive phobia in Japan, in some ways resembling social phobia in DSM-IV. This syndrome refers to an individual's intense fear that his or her body, its parts or its functions, displease, embarrass, or are offensive to other people in appearance, odor, facial expressions, or movements. This syndrome is included in the official Japanese diagnostic system for mental disorders.

Zar—A general term applied in Ethiopia, Somalia, Egypt, Sudan, Iran, and other North African and Middle Eastern societies to the experience of spirits possessing an individual. Persons possessed by a spirit may experience dissociative episodes that may include shouting, laughing, hitting the head against a wall, singing, or weeping. Individuals may show apathy and withdrawal, refusing to eat or carry out daily tasks, or may develop a long-term relationship with the possessing spirit. Such behavior is not considered pathological locally.

Source: American Psychiatric Association. (2000). *Diagnostic and statistical manual of mental disorders* (Revised 4th ed., Text Revision). Washington, DC: American Psychiatric Association.

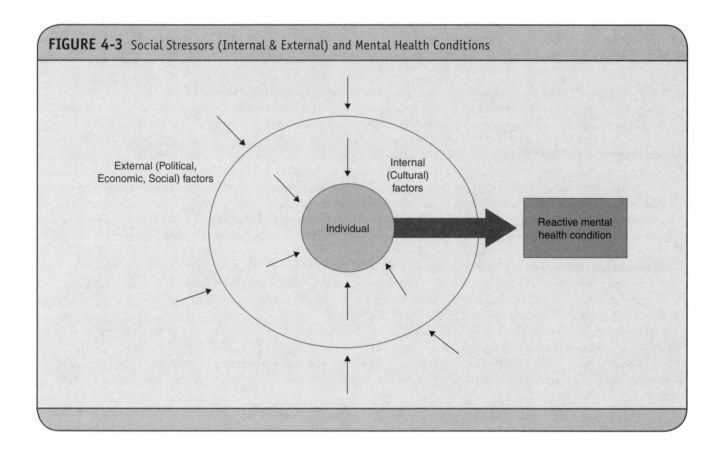

FIGURE 4-3 Social Stressors (Internal & External) and Mental Health Conditions

Here are five interesting examples of how this might work:

Stress Response in the Saora of India

Some sources have reported a peculiar condition (a "shamanic initiatory illness") among young men and women in the Saora tribe in India (O'Neil 2008). They cry and laugh at inappropriate times, experience memory loss, pass out, and feel like they are bitten by ants when no ants are present. The youth that express this condition seem to be teenagers or young adults who are, in a sense, misfits. They are apparently not interested in pursuing the traditional subsistence farming life. For this, they are under considerable psychological stress due to social pressure from relatives and friends. The Saora themselves explain this behavior as caused by the actions of supernatural beings who want to marry the youth. To resolve the problem, a marriage ceremony is carried out in which the disturbed person is married to the spirit. Following the marriage, the abnormal symptoms apparently end

and the young person becomes a shaman responsible for curing people. This represents a very interesting transformation, where the youth begin as misfits but have a culturally ritualized way out that ultimately results in positive gain—the Saora gain an additional shaman, who is valuable, respected, and legitimized by his/her contact with the supernatural. In this case, the disturbed (mental health) condition could be seen as a coping mechanism in an otherwise difficult social predicament (ibid.).

Anfechtung among the Hutterites of Canada

The Hutterites are a Christian, Anabaptist group similar to the Amish and Mennonites in North America. They speak a dialect of German, and live in closed communities where all property is communally owned. Hutterite children were traditionally educated within the community, though in recent years they have attended public schools—in part because of the technological needs of maintaining the large agricultural operations characteristic of these communities. Like similar groups, the Hutterites are also firmly pacifist (Janzen & Stanton 2010). Religious services are an important part of daily life, and the religious and governing structures are the same. The condition of *Anfechtung* is a kind of psychosis in which the victim experiences intense guilt, anxiety, and depression over having been conflicted about temptation—in other words, guilt because of spiritual conflict or insufficient faith. It is not viewed as a secular illness or disease, and it is treated by surrounding the victim with caring community members, prayer, and repeated visits from a preacher. The victim also needs to ask for forgiveness. When the disruptive spiritual conflict is resolved, the illness symptoms go away. Thinking about the cultural context, it could be that the condition is a reaction to pressures inherent in the communal living and social expectation of faith.

Anorexia/Bulimia (Eating Disorders) in the United States

These disorders primarily affect adolescent females in the United States (and Western European countries to some degree), although in some cases males have also been affected. Basically, *anorexia nervosa* refers to an extreme fear of weight gain and a distorted view of one's actual body size. This causes young people to restrict their eating by severe dieting, fasting, and/or exercise, and sometimes by binge eating followed by purging (using laxatives or something that will induce vomiting). It can cause serious health problems, and over time, a person with this condition becomes very thin and frail. A related but very different eating disorder is *bulimia nervosa*, which involves a regular pattern of binge eating and purging, by forced vomiting and laxatives. Again, it is related to a fear of weight gain. At least one of the key contributing factors is the combination of normal weight gain during puberty set against perceived social pressure to conform to culturally specific, ideal standards of beauty and body type represented by models and celebrities who are very thin—even stick-like—and

FIGURE 4-4 Hutterite Family

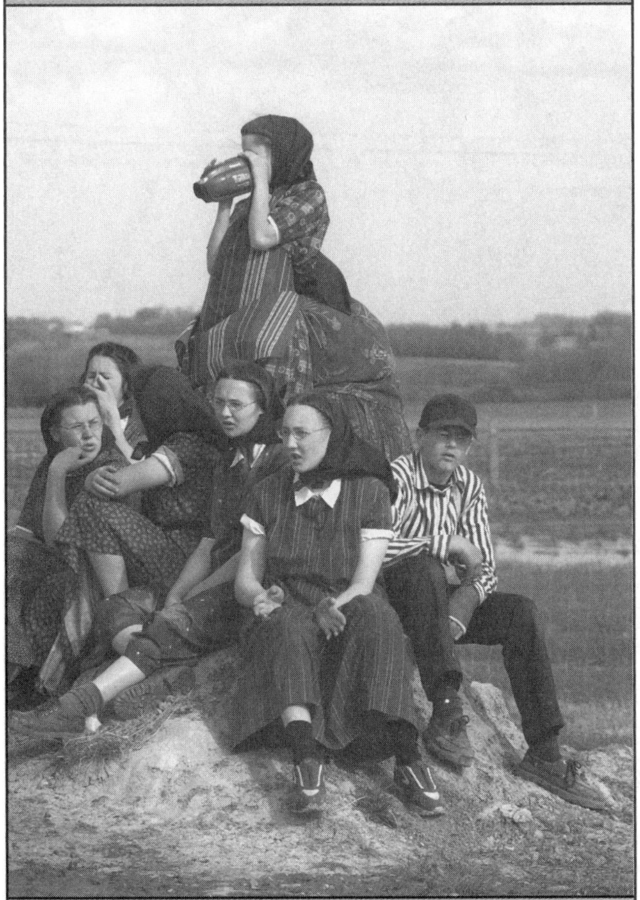

Source: © Jack Dagley Photography/ShutterStock, Inc.

FIGURE 4-5 Model Isabelle Caro—Anorexia Victim who Died at Age 28

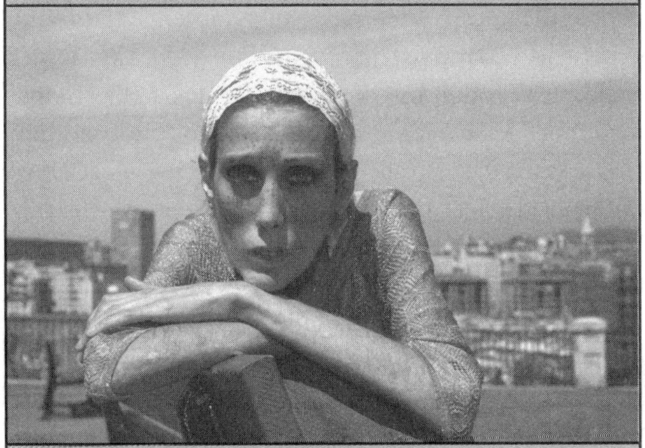

Source: © Mercier Serge/Maxppp/Landov

whose photos and pictures seem to be everywhere, in magazines, ads, on the Internet, social media, television, and in any other media. Yet being thin and stick-like is *not* the ideal of feminine beauty everywhere in the world (see, for example, *Eating Disorders*, accessed through the National Institute of Mental Health, at www.nimh.nih.gov/health/publications/ eating-disorders/complete-index.shtml, and Steiner & Lock 1998).

Historical Trauma among American Indian Populations

American Indian/Alaska Native (AI/AN) populations have long experienced a range of disparities in health: AI/ANs die from diabetes at a rate almost twice that of Caucasians, and coronary heart disease rates are very high (U.S. DHHS 2005a and 2005b; Howard et al. 1999; Rhoades 2005). Why are the risks for these and other health conditions so high for many AI/AN populations? There are a lot of factors that have been associated with health disparities in general. But one factor that has been identified as a possible contributor, at a deeper level, among AI/AN peoples is referred to as *historical trauma*—a collective, psychological scar resulting from the experience of violence, culture loss, land loss, discrimination, and eventual marginalization that resulted from European colonialism and conquest in the Americas (Brave Heart 1999; Brave Heart & DeBruyn 1998; Brave Heart-Jordan 1995). Duran et al. (1999) have referred to historical trauma as a "soul wound."

This scar, or soul wound that is felt by many AI/AN people includes a wide range of symptoms and living experiences. Perceived discrimination, depression, loss of self-esteem, conditions of poverty, and loss of traditional male roles have been cited as aspects of the condition (Rhoades 2003; also see Oetting et al. 1998). A sense of unresolved grief from historical trauma (Brave Heart & DeBruyn, 1998) is another way of framing how people feel; particularly among younger men, there is a feeling of aimlessness/rootlessness (anomie) and a loss of cultural identity (O'Nell & Mitchell, 1996). Recent research has attempted to clarify the cause of these symptoms through the use of a historical loss scale (Whitbeck et al. 2004) and the emotions that result as reported in an historical loss associated symptoms scale. The key is that there is a

shared psychological phenomenon resulting from conditions particular to AI/AN peoples.

Immigrant/Refugee Mental Health Syndromes

Many immigrant and refugee populations coming to the United States and other host countries from civil wars, disasters, and other traumatic situations experience psychological consequences in addition to the stress of acculturation itself. Mental health problems, for example, are very prevalent among Central American immigrants and include high rates of posttraumatic stress disorder, depres-

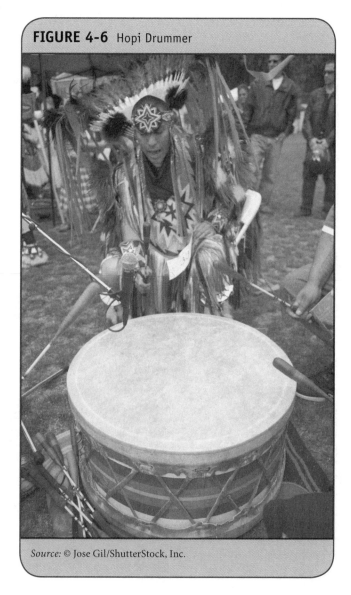

FIGURE 4-6 Hopi Drummer

Source: © Jose Gil/ShutterStock, Inc.

sion, and panic disorder (Eisenman et al. 2003) directly attributable to the experience of political violence and even torture prior to immigration to the United States. Similar mental health issues have affected refugees and immigrants from Ethiopia, many of whom also went through various kinds of traumatic situations before emigrating, followed by refugee camp internment and then adjustment difficulties in the host country (Fenta, Hyman, & Noh, 2004). One study of Somali and Ethiopian (Oromo ethnic group) refugees in Minnesota identified an experience of torture prevalence ranging from 25% to 69% with women being tortured as often as men, and torture survivors having more health problems including posttraumatic stress syndrome (Jaranson et al. 2004).

Once these immigrants and refuges arrive in a host country, it is often difficult to adjust. Social status and gender roles, for example, may be very different. Where an immigrant held a position of high status in the home country, that position may not mean anything in the new setting. Or where males were household authorities and breadwinners in the home country, that may also be turned on its head in the host country because it is often easier for women to find immediate or short-term work. Family lines of authority can also be disrupted, with children learning the new language more quickly and serving as information brokers, even to their parents. All of these can produce a range of psychological consequences, including depression, substance abuse, and

FIGURE 4-7 Refugee Camp in Sudan

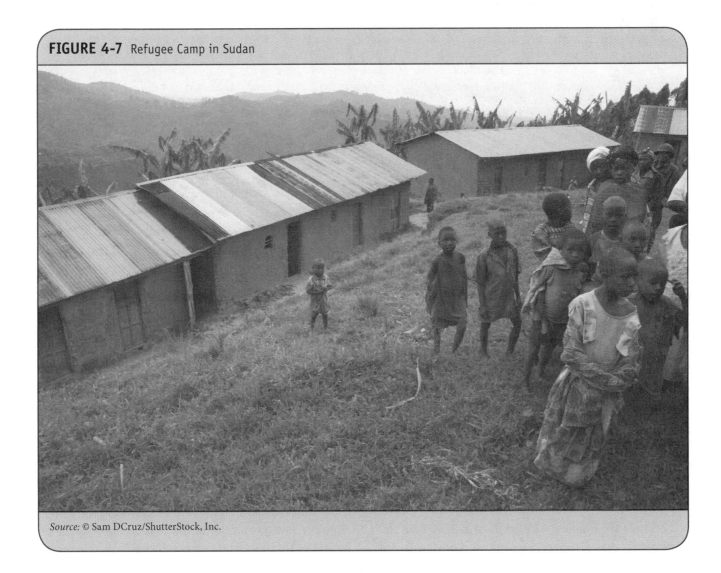

Source: © Sam DCruz/ShutterStock, Inc.

EXHIBIT 4-1 Diagnosing Laura . . .

Let's say that the healer described in Chapter 1 is taking all the symptoms that he sees in Laura Smith—both the physical and emotional symptoms—as representing a general condition that is a kind of somatized (expressed physically) psychological phenomenon. Consider the following:

- She does have physical symptoms—the nausea, apparent fever, physical pain in her side, and feet.
- Emotionally, she seems to be aggravated and slightly unbalanced, veering from distrust and impatience to straightforward responses to his questions, then back to impatience.
- She is highly directional; she seems bent on pursuing a particular path and set of activities that are all linked up with other activities and goals, like graduate school, management, and so on. To the healer, this seems like a complex web of control behavior.

He has seen this before. Not so much among people from his own country and culture, but among Westerners. Some of them just seem to be in a hurry and get thrown into a loop if their lists and plans and linked activities are disturbed in some way. But to the healer, disturbance and change, are just normal—natural, if you will.

He scratches his chin. *I think that this Laura Smith has what I call dominance-control syndrome. I have talked about this with some of my fellow practitioners who have treated people from Western countries. You, know, the belief that the natural world is inside a box of some kind, operated by buttons. They can just push a button here, another there, and get what they want. And when something goes wrong, they get flustered and aggravated, as if their world is broken for no reason they can discern. These emotions go through their body like a wave, and they start feeling all kinds of pains they can't explain. Yes, that's it. I'll give her some teas for her nausea and a meditation stick. If she can just focus on the meditation stick, it will take her thinking away from this world in a box for at least a little bit, and restore her equilibrium, her body balance.*

Ah, but . . . I don't know if she'll listen to me. I am (he chuckles) just a native, eh? No white coat. Well, I can try . . .

family stress, that form a pattern not uncommon among different refugee and immigrant populations.

EMOTIONS AND CULTURE

How about emotions? Are they universal to all peoples or are they unique? Although much research has pointed to the connection between basic human genetic makeup and emotions (see, for example, Sauter and colleague's 2010 study), some scholars and researchers have a different view. The anthropologist Catherine Lutz (1988), argued that emotions themselves are culturally constructed—not universal—and that particular emotional patterns vary across societies. In her well-known book, *Unnatural Emotions* (Lutz 1988), she uses her work among the Ifaluk people (Western Pacific Islander) to demonstrate the way in which emotions are not biologically determined, but culturally constructed. Western thinking about emotion is shaped by several philosophical positions. According to Lutz (1988):

- There is a dualism in Western thought about the mind that separates thought (cognition) from emotion, where emotion is the lesser and weaker partner and genderized as female.
- There is a belief in psychic unity, where emotions are viewed as cross-cultural constants.
- Emotions have names that frame them as "objectivized internal event-things" (pp. 9) that are primarily physical in nature. This mirrors the general American linguistic pattern of viewing language as primarily referential and labeling in function, rather than constructive and pragmatic.
- Emotions are constructed as wild and of nature, rather than of culture, and as such are less controllable and less accountable.
- Emotions are subjective, not objective.

By contrast, Lutz argues that emotions are culturally constructed. They are, she says, pragmatic, not just referential. In other words, emotions are a daily-life working phenomenon. To talk about emotions is to talk about the things that are meaningful in a society or local culture, because emotions are a marker and a consequence of the things that are intensely meaningful. In this sense, emotions are discourse; that is, language and symbolic communication that encapsulate culture.

The Ifaluk live on an atoll in the Pacific island chain known as the Federated States of Micronesia. Ifaluk is remote, and traditional ways of living are maintained to a large degree. Fish and taro (a root) are primary food sources.

Lutz spent a considerable amount of time conducting ethnographic research there, recording natural discourse about emotion very carefully. She concluded that the range of emotions expressed by Ifaluk are connected to Ifaluk values, of which a central value is social intelligence. This is essentially a deep understanding about social roles and relations, cohesiveness, and the importance of cooperation for Ifaluk life. A person cannot attain social intelligence until he or she is about 6 or 7 years old, and leaders or highly respected persons will have a well-developed sense of this. Many Ifaluk emotions are related to social intelligence. Here is a selected list:

- *Fago:* Translated as a combination of love, compassion, and sadness. According to Lutz, this is a key emotional construct for the Ifaluk. It can be felt as admiration or love for someone (for a child, a spouse, admiration for a chief, admiration when someone exhibits exemplary behavior, etc.), as compassion, when others are sick or in need—of nurturance, which is equally valued for men and women, says Lutz—and as sadness (crying big) due to death or absence/loss of kin.[1]

- *Maluwelu:* Translated as calmness—a key emotional state in Ifaluk society, according to Lutz.
- *Song:* Translated as justifiable anger, resulting from a moral or interpersonal offense.
- *Ma:* Translated as shame or embarrassment.
- *Sig:* Translated as being angry in the more general sense, as distinct from *song*.
- *Metagu* and *rus:* These are translated as fear and panic/fright/surprise (in combination)—from encounters with spirits, unfamiliar people, interpersonal violence, physical injury, and death (as from typhoons). It is, according to Lutz, related to a sense that existence is precarious.
- *Ker:* Translated as the combination of happy/excited, which can spill over into improper actions.

Now we come to the pragmatic part in Lutz's argument. Basically, life is very vulnerable in Ifaluk. The highest part of the island is a mere few meters above sea level, so typhoons and other storms can be very dangerous, and there is no quick way to travel from Ifaluk to other islands or atolls. So, in Lutz's argument, it has historically been extremely important for the Ifaluk to be collaborative and maintain good social cohesion. This is the root of social intelligence and the emotions that surround it—to promote the kinds of social relations that are necessary for survival. From this perspective, Ifaluk emotions are a creation of Ifaluk society and its practical needs, not biologically determined phenomena. More important (to Lutz's argument), because these emotions are directly related to the Ifaluk environment, they are, more or less, unique to the Ifaluk and not generic or common to all people.

---

[1] There is a relationship between *fago* and power—those who are the objects of *fago* (except when it is expressed as admiration) are often those who are most vulnerable, most in need. In order to feel the emotion of *fago*, one must have social intelligence—so, those who are the most socially intelligent (mature adults, chiefs) are most capable of the full range of *fago*.

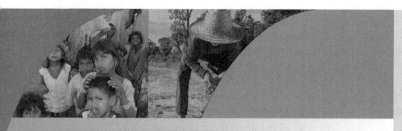

QUESTIONS

1. Can you think of any mental health conditions that seem to be specific to American or European societies? What do you think are the social pressures/forces that have contributed to such conditions?

2. What is your position? Are emotions and mental health conditions the same for all peoples, just called by different names (psychic unity view)? Or are they unique based on culture (cultural relativist view)?

3. With what kind of ethnomedical system would the culture-reactive syndrome (in the DSM-IV list) called *rootwork* most likely be associated?

4. With what kind of ethnomedical system would *qi-gong syndrome* (in the DSM-IV list) most likely be associated?

5. With what kind of ethnomedical system would *susto* (in the DSM-IV list) most likely be associated? (Hint: This one is a little more complicated.)

REFERENCES

American Psychiatric Association. 2000. *Diagnostic and Statistical Manual of Mental Disorders*, Revised 4th ed. (Text Revision). Arlington, VA: American Psychiatric Publishing, Inc.

Brave Heart, M.Y.H. 1999. "Oyate Ptayela: Rebuilding the Lakota Nation through Addressing Historical Trauma among Lakota Parents." *Journal of Human Behavior in the Social Environment* 2 (1–2): 109–126.

Brave Heart, M.Y.H., and L.M. DeBruyn. 1998. "The American Indian Holocaust: Healing Historical Unresolved Grief." *American Indian and Alaska Native Mental Health Research* 8 (2): 56–78.

Brave Heart-Jordan, M.Y.H. 1995. *The Return to the Sacred Path: Healing from Historical Trauma and Historical Unresolved Grief among the Lakota*. Unpublished doctoral dissertation. Smith College, Northampton, MA.

Cartwright, S.A. 1851. "Report on the Diseases and Physical Peculiarities of the Negro Race," *The New Orleans Medical and Surgical Journal* 1851: 691–715.

Chinese Association of Psychiatry. 1995. *Chinese Classification of Mental Disorders (CCMD-2-R)*. Southeast University Press, Nanjing.

De Ramirez, R.D., and E.S. Shapiro. 2005. "Effects of Student Ethnicity on Judgments of ADHD Symptoms among Hispanic and White Teachers." *School Psychology Quarterly* 20(3): 268–287.

Duran, B., E. Duran, and M.Y.H. Brave Heart. 1999. "Native Americans and the Trauma of History." In *Studying Native America: Problems and Prospects*, edited by R. Thornton. Madison, WI: University of Wisconsin Press.

Eisenman, D. P., L. Gelberg, L. Honghu, and M. Shapiro. 2003. "Mental Health and Health-Related Quality of Life among Adult Latino Primary Care Patients Living in the United States with Previous Exposure to Political Violence." *JAMA* 290 (5): 627–634.

Fenta, H., I. Hyman, and S. Noh. 2004. "Determinants of Depression among Ethiopian Immigrants and Refugees in Toronto. *Journal of Nervous and Mental Disorders* 192 (5): 363–372.

Howard, B.V., E.T. Lee, L.D. Cowan, R.B. Devereux, J.M. Galloway, O.T. Go, W.J. Howard, E.R. Rhoades, D.C. Robbins, M.L. Sievers, and T.K. Welty. 1999. "Rising Tide of Cardiovascular Disease in American Indians. The Strong Heart Study." *Circulation*, 99 (18): 2389–2395.

Hughes, C.C. 1998. "The Glossary of Culture-Bound Syndromes in DSM-IV: A Critique." *Transcultural Psychiatry* 35: 413.

Janzen, R., and M. Stanton. 2010. *The Hutterites in North America*. Baltimore, MD: Johns Hopkins University Press.

Jaranson, J. M., J. Butcher, L. Halcon, D. R. Johnson, C. Robertson, K., Savik, M. Spring, and J. Westermeyer. 2004. "Somali and Oromo Refugees: Correlates of Torture and Trauma History." *American Journal of Public Health* 94 (4): 591–598.

Lutz, C.A. 1988. *Unnatural Emotions: Everyday Sentiments on a Micronesian Atoll and Their Challenge to Western Theory*. Chicago: University of Chicago Press.

Oetting, E.R., J.F. Donnermeyer, J.E. Trimble, and F. Beauvais. 1998. "Primary Socialization Theory: Culture, Ethnicity, and Cultural Identification. The Links between Culture and Substance Use. IV." *Substance Use & Misuse* 33 (10): 2075–2107.

O'Neil, D. Updated 2008. *Medical Anthropology: How Illness is Traditionally Perceived and Cured Around the World—Culture-Specific Diseases*. San Marcos, CA: Palomar College, Behavioral Sciences Department, website, accessed at http://anthro.palomar.edu/medical/default.htm.

O'Nell, T.D., and C.M. Mitchell. 1996. "Alcohol Use among American Indian Adolescents: The role of Culture in Pathological Drinking." *Social Science & Medicine* 42 (4): 565–578.

Parker, S.P. 2003. *McGraw-Hill Dictionary of Scientific and Technical Terms (6th Edition)*. New York: McGraw Hill.

Puig, M., M.C. Lambert, G.T. Rowan, T. Winfrey, M. Lyubansky, S. Hannah, and M. Hill. 1999. "Behavioral and Emotional Problems among Jamaican and African-American Children, Ages 6–11: Teacher Reports versus Direct Observations." *Journal of Emotional and Behavioral Disorders* 7: 240–250.

Rhoades, D.A. 2005. "Racial Misclassification and Disparities in Cardiovascular Disease among American Indians and Alaska Natives." *Circulation* 111 (10): 1250–1256.

Rhoades, E.R. 2003. "The Health Status of American Indian and Alaska Native Males." *American Journal of Public Health* 93(5): 774–778.

Sauter, D.A., F. Eisner, P. Ekman, and S.K. Scott. 2010. "Cross-Cultural Recognition of Basic Emotions Through Non-Verbal Emotional Vocalizations." *Proceedings of the National Academy of Sciences* 107 (6): 2408–2412.

Simons, R.C., and C.C. Hughes, eds. 1985. *The Culture-Bound Syndromes: Folk Illnesses of Psychological and Anthropological Interest*. Dordrecht, The Netherlands: S. Reidel.

Steiner, H., and J. Lock. 1998. "Anorexia Nervosa and Bulimia Nervosa in Children and Adolescents: A Review of the Past Ten Years." *Journal of the American Academy of Child and Adolescent Psychiatry* 37: 352–359.

U.S. Department of Health and Human Services. 1999. *Mental Health: A Report of the Surgeon General*. Rockville, MD: U.S. Department of Health and Human Services, Substance Abuse and Mental Health Services Administration, Center for Mental Health Services, National Institutes of Health, National Institute of Mental Health.

U. S. Department of Health and Human Services. 2005a. *Behavioral Risk Factor Surveillance System Survey Data*. Atlanta, GA: Centers for Disease Control and Prevention.

U. S. Department of Health and Human Services. 2005b. *Health, United States, 2005, With Chartbook on Trends in the Health of Americans*. Washington, DC: DHHS.

Weisz, J.R., W. Chaiyasit, B. Weiss, K.L. Eastman, and E.W. Jackson. 1995. "Multimethod Study of Problem Behavior among Thai and American Children in School: Teacher Reports versus Direct Observations." *Child Development* 66: 402–415.

Whitbeck, L.B., G.W. Adams, D.R. Hoyt, and X. Chen. 2004. "Conceptualizing and Measuring Historical Trauma among American Indian People." *American Journal of Community Psychology* 33 (3/4): 119–130.

Winkelman, M. 2009. *Culture and Health: Applying Medical Anthropology*. San Francisco, CA: Jossey-Bass.

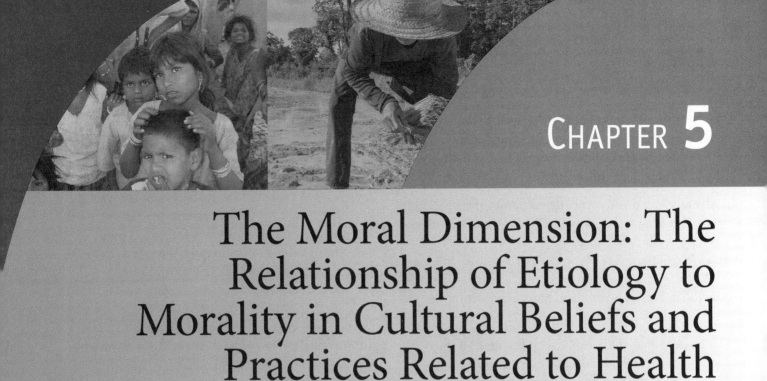

CHAPTER 5

The Moral Dimension: The Relationship of Etiology to Morality in Cultural Beliefs and Practices Related to Health

"Having good health is very different from only being not sick."

—Seneca the Younger (Roman Stoic philosopher, approximately 3 BCE–65 ACE)

Following through with other implications of cultural systems of health knowledge, belief, and practice—ethnomedical systems—there is also a moral dimension that plays a very important role in the social impact of illness. This dimension illustrates very vividly the intersection between cultural values and health and one aspect of the social construction of illness. Recall that an ethnomedical system involves a linkage between types of illnesses, their causes, and appropriate treatments. We have also seen, in our discussion so far, that cross-cultural etiologies (causes) of illness can range from those that seem neutral, like pathogens and genetics, to those that don't, like sorcery or family disharmony. In other words, there appear to be some causes for which no judgment can be made or blame assigned, and some that can be blamed on somebody or something, whether the person who is ill, or another person, or another social institution or group. That is very much because culture, as reflected in ethnomedical systems, involves socially produced definitions of what is normal vs. not normal (well described by social

philosophers such as Michel Foucault 1975; 1979; 1980), good vs. bad, and so on. These kinds of judgmental categories, for the most part, come to exist below the level of conscious thought. They are naturalized. They are also routinized in the language used, and the way people talk about such matters. So when a person experiences some abnormal, illness phenomenon, it could be thought of as:

- Abnormal but morally OK = Not your fault
- Abnormal but not morally OK = Your fault or somebody's fault. Importantly, this can result in stigma (we'll discuss this later in the chapter)

As for most of the culture–health relationships we cover in this book, these vary across cultures and societies, though there are some patterns that have been consistent. The moral connection to illness is very much related to several kinds of factors:

- Cultural conceptions of the individual and the degree to which individuals are viewed as responsible for their condition and their behavior.
- The degree to which external forces are viewed as responsible for a person's condition and/or behavior.
- The kinds of social divisions that exist in a particular society and what those social divisions are held

to mean—social class/social stratification, gender, race/ethnicity, religion, and other divisions.

- The physical symbolism of the disease itself—how a particular culture interprets this and reacts.

All of these can lead to the *stigmatization* of people with a particular illness or disease. Let's look at each of these factors in a little more depth.

Individuals, Circumstances and Behavior. We may take for granted many things about the idea of an individual, but, as noted in a companion text on health behavior (Edberg 2007):

> You may think this is a no-brainer. An individual is, just like me, you say, an autonomous self that has a distinct physical unity (me, my body and I), a personality, a way of talking, a way of walking, my own goals, my own motivations, and the ability to plan, initiate carry out action. You know, ME. . . . but let's just look at that for a second. We can start with that body of yours. Your physical being, as you know, is genetic—it comes from parents and other ancestors. So, yes, it's you, but, it's kind of them too. Now let's go to that personality. Some of that may have genetic influences too. But your personality, your way of talking, walking, dressing, and all that . . . you didn't think all of that up from scratch, did you? You got it from somewhere. Just like the musician who is called a "unique" sax player, you pulled together pieces of "how to be," kind of like those riffs on the sax. You put them together in your own way. But most of those pieces didn't magically appear. They came from the social and cultural world around you, including your family; the examples of "how to be male" or "how to be female" that you saw in your personal life, on television, videos or film; from the tales, stories, songs and other narratives about people who were good versus people who were not; what a good life consists of; lessons and advice from family, community, faith organizations; people you have seen who have a style

or a "look" that you like and want to emulate; and so on!

> It's not so easy to draw a clear line between yourself and everyone else. Of course you take all these influences and shape them, "inhabit" them as your individual life. Yet this process inexorably connects you to your world, and complicates easy descriptions of individual behavior and motivation." (ibid., 36)

There is a wide variety in the way different cultures "put the onus" on individuals. Most Western societies are typically viewed as individual-centric, compared, for example, to Asian and other cultures. The French anthropologist Louis Dumont (1986, 1980)—among others—highlighted a distinction between societies said to be constructed of individuals (an individual is the basic, autonomous unit) and those in which individuals are seen as an outcome of society, and where society or major social units such as the family may be viewed as more important than individuals. His distinction between *societas* and *universitas* refers to the idea of societies that result from individuals who decide to associate (*societas*) versus societies that are viewed at a higher level, where individuals are just reflections of that society (*universitas*). Much of the discourse about health in the United States, for example, has been much more likely to use the terms *individual responsibility* and personal *lifestyle* when talking about the causes of various illnesses. As a result, individuals are more likely to be blamed for the health problems they experience.

External Forces, Circumstances, and Behavior. It is hard to resist using the comedian's phrase "the devil made me do it" here, because—apart from its comedic use—it says a lot about another kind of cultural position on general causality. In many cultures, what you do and what happens to you may not originate with you, but with other forces. These forces could be attributed to one or more gods, to broader natural forces, to specific spirits, or to sorcery and witchcraft. For example, studies on attitudes and beliefs about cancer have found that, among different Latino populations (see, for example, Collins et al. 2008; Chavez et al. 1999), it is not uncommon to believe that a person has cancer as a consequence of having done something bad or immoral, and that the outcome of cancer treatment is up to God, or simply that whatever happens is due to the will of God. This particular attitude has sometimes been referred to as "fatalistic." People from an animist culture—e.g., in the rural or remote areas of Southeast Asia—might say that a person became ill because he or she angered or disturbed the spirit of a tree, or a stream, whether on purpose or by accident. Many studies of HIV/AIDS in Africa have pointed to beliefs related to sorcery as the cause (see, for example, Mshana et al. 2006 regarding Tanzania; Thomas 2007 regarding Namibia), or at least a willingness to employ allegations of sorcery and witchcraft. So, in these cases, an individual may be blamed for his condition if he did something to trigger the action from the external source, or he may not have had anything to do with it and so would not be blamed. The moral source, so to speak, may in part be related to individuals, but indirectly.

Social Divisions, Circumstances, and Behavior. This is an entire area related to the etiology of disease/illness that we will get into in much more detail later, in Chapter 7. Basically, this refers to a moral source that is society itself—the way in which a society creates conditions that make some people more vulnerable to disease than others, or that forces some people into choices (with health consequences) that others do not have to make. Think for a minute about the famous quote by 19th century French novelist and journalist Anatole France: "The law, in its majestic equality, forbids rich and poor alike to sleep under bridges, to beg in the streets, and to steal bread" (from *The Red Lily*, 1894). Who, of course, will be affected by this law? The issue of culture and morality here focuses on the question of who is to blame when people are ill because of socially created vulnerabilities. Is it the individuals? Is it an external source of some kind? Or is it the social and political arrangements themselves, and those who benefit from them?

This is all complicated by the fact that social divisions are often naturalized (made to seem natural) through cultural beliefs. If individuals who are poor and vulnerable are seen via a particular set of beliefs to be primarily responsible for their condition because of personal or moral weakness in some way, then their social position becomes justified. If the social hierarchy is explained through a cultural belief in the divine or

spiritual superiority of specific social classes, then those on the lower levels of the social order may be understood to be inferior and therefore their vulnerability to disease not as important (see Singer 2008 for an excellent discussion of this issue concerning illegal drug use and abuse). Social hierarchies and their cultural justifications may also be based on gender distinctions, on racialized or ethnic categories, or on other characteristics. In any case, one way to look at moral judgment with respect to causes of disease is at the societal level, where these social divisions contribute to who gets sick and who doesn't. One of the clearest examples of this, across a number of societies, concerns HIV/AIDS. While moral judgments are often made about AIDS victims, it is largely the case that most victims come from social groups that are more vulnerable to begin with because of their social position, which in itself creates high risks for exposure.

The Physical Symbolism of the Disease. Sometimes, in addition to or exclusive of the other moral dimensions already mentioned, something about the physical appearance of disease symptoms may play into fears and the popular imaginary. The disease itself symbolizes something. This has certainly been the case with leprosy (see "Leprosy [Hansen's Disease]: The Classic Case of Stigma," later in this chapter), and it could be with other diseases as well, where a person appears wasted and ghostlike, or develops severe tumors or other physical anomalies. If the appearance of the disease *looks* like the embodiment of a culturally defined malevolence of some kind, people may react to it regardless of whether or not the victim is initially held to be at fault. Alternatively, the appearance of the disease may seem like evidence that the person *must be* at fault or in some way selected for punishment, triggering a kind of after-the-fact blame.

STIGMA

The profound result of moral judgments applied to illnesses is *stigma*—the discrediting, social rejection or staining of types of people who are viewed as blameworthy in one way or another. The sociologist Erving Goffman (1963) referred to stigma as the social construction of spoiled identity for classes of people viewed as undesirable by some social standard. A stigmatized individual or class of individuals is typically shunned, shamed, excluded, and subject to abuse of many kinds—and this is viewed as acceptable because of their specific status. The exclusion and abuse may even be sanctioned by law. This is the end product of the moral issues raised so far. When cultural beliefs related to illness and its causes lead to judgment and blame, those individuals or groups are stigmatized. As we will see in the discussion about leprosy and HIV/AIDS, stigma creates a barrier that is often difficult to overcome when trying to work with or address affected individuals or groups with health promotion and prevention efforts. Understanding its roots may help.

ILLNESS BEHAVIOR

Remember one of the definitional types for culture (in Chapter 2) that cast culture as a kind of theatrical play in which members of the culture, more or less, know the script? That particular definition is very much in evidence in considering what people do in any culture when they are ill, or when others are ill. What people do is very much entwined with how the illness is understood in a moral sense. For that reason, behavior related to illness can be seen as coded or symbolic behavior because it represents how the illness is viewed. Staying with the same theatrical analogy, within a particular culture there are sick roles that "script" behavior based on people's expectations about how their particular illness is viewed. Let's break it down. There are two kinds of sick roles in this grand play:

1. A set of roles for people who are ill
2. A set of roles for the other people who interact with the sick person, whether as a healer or family member or even a classmate

Think of this scenario: a person named Jack Sullivan comes down with a flulike illness. Jack is a hard-working, solid person who is very responsible. He is not known for living life on the edge, or being unpredictable, or for really any excess at all. So when he gets sick, others around him do not think he is at fault, and they sympathize with how he is feeling, offer to help him, and his boss just tells him, "Go ahead, take a couple of days off, Jack. You deserve it." Jack doesn't believe he did anything wrong to deserve being sick either. He thinks to himself,

"Well, I must have caught it from somewhere. That just happens sometimes." He appreciates when people offer to help take care of some of his work if he takes off—and they do. He goes home and relaxes on his couch. His wife brings him some tea and a blanket, and he doesn't answer his phone messages. No one has a problem with this; in fact, they expect it.

On the other hand, there is Jack's cousin Marvin.

Marvin does a good job at work, too. But Marvin is different. People are a little unsure about him. Sometimes he comes in late, with a generally scruffy appearance including messed-up hair. He wears shoes that are a little too loud in terms of taste. He stays out late and is known to go to clubs and get a little wild. He will sometimes ask people to do him a favor or lend him some money, for reasons people don't quite understand. He just can't sustain a relationship either; he has been divorced twice and everyone at work hears about it. When he gets the flu, the reaction is a little different than it is with Jack. The lady at the front desk shakes her head and says "Marvin, that's what you get when you live life like you do." Others around the office smirk behind his back. No one offers to take over any of his work, and the boss doesn't suggest that he take a day off. Yet Marvin thinks to himself, "Hey, I'm sick. I need a day off. I'm going to ask. I mean, anyone who's sick deserves a day off." The boss doesn't give it to him.

Why doesn't Marvin get the day off? Why don't people help him with his work? Because they blame him for his illness. He has the same illness as Jack does, but something about his behavior violates moral codes and changes the script. Marvin could respond by getting angry at his coworkers' lack of sympathy, but if he does he will violate the code further, because as a morally suspect sick person, he shouldn't be demanding that others treat him as if he were blameless. If he wants to abide by the general script for this, he should be quiet, not ask anybody for anything, and slink away at the end of the day and go home and take care of himself. In other words, he should act as a symbol of what his illness represents. If he does this, he might actually get some sympathy at some point because he will be acting according to the script.

There are many other scenarios that illustrate the same point. In a culture with a male gender concept in which males are not to call for help when the situation is not really serious, the available script for behavior when a man thinks he is ill would be to hold it in, tough it out, or something similar, but *not* to go get medical help—unless of course, something very obvious and serious happens. If a man does go for medical help when it is not justified under this code, he may be judged as having a weak character, or being less than a man.

Culturally coded illness behavior may also affect patient–healer interaction. On one project assessing barriers to accessing care at clinics/providers serving people with limited English-speaking skills, the author and an evaluation team encountered issues facing older Chinese women when they accessed doctors who were Chinese, and where one would think barriers to care would be lower. However, gender issues and their impact on illness

behavior got in the way. The Chinese doctors, it seemed, often brushed off health complaints by older women as female griping, and were not receptive when women asked them questions (as the intervention program encouraged them to do). Women faced a culturally based role that prohibited them from questioning a male authority figure such as a doctor. The scripted sick role was to quietly listen to what the doctor said and then follow his instructions. Some doctors were apparently unhappy when their female patients violated this role.

Illness Behavior and Culture. Thinking about these scripts, it is easy to see that illness behavior is produced or socially constructed within the framework of a culture. It involves an entire production, in which many players act out their roles and in doing so, work together to produce a result that comes out as the way a particular illness takes form, and the consequences of that, in a given society. An important result of this and other culturally shaped interactions is to reproduce the culture. In fact, it wouldn't be a stretch to say that culture is reproduced through the aggregate impact of many of these little productions, linked together. In playing out a role,

---

BOX 5-1 Laura Smith and Illness Behavior

Some of the confusion and concern that Laura experienced in the introductory scenario in Chapter 1 had everything to do with illness behavior and scripts. She, of course, was used to a certain patient–doctor script and was uncomfortable when that script did not unfold. Not only that, but here was this strange healer, bringing up her lifestyle, her ambitions, and, well . . . using that in his discussion about her ailment! You can imagine what she might have been thinking. . . . *What kind of questions are these? What is he thinking? He's not supposed to do that, and in any case, it has nothing to do with my stomach problem! And . . . it even sounds a little like he's blaming me, you know, something about how I am, for what is wrong here! I mean, it's a germ, or bacteria or something. Bacteria don't care if I am in a hurry all the time or whether or not I have an internship! That's like, ridiculous! Makes me mad, too.*

Oh what a relief she felt when she found the clinic that looked, smelled, and functioned like the script she knew!

Okay, so the doctor did ask if I drank too much or used any drugs or anything. But I get that. There's a medical reason for it. I'm so glad I found an actual doctor! She certainly didn't ask me about what I wanted to do or how much of a hurry I am in, or any of that. It's just not medical. It's out of bounds, you know.

EXHIBIT 5-1 Arthur Kleinman and Illness Narratives

Arthur Kleinman, MD, Esther and Sidney Rabb Professor of Anthropology at Harvard and former chair of the Department of Social Medicine, is a pioneering medical anthropologist and psychiatrist whose work has shaped the dialog about the cross-cultural experience and meaning of illness. His work has contributed greatly to the understanding of Chinese and East Asian culture-specific illnesses, and one of his other major contributions has concerned illness narratives and on social suffering related to the way in which illness is culturally constructed (see Kleinman 1988; Kleinman, Das, & Lock 1997). Illness narratives refer to the way that patients, in their social and cultural contexts, experience and talk about illness and its effect on them, and its implications for their social worlds. In so doing, patients embed their experience in the cultural meanings attached to the illness, including the stigma, suffering, and daily indignities (or dignities) that they face.

people participate in the reproduction of their culturally shaped experience of health. That is one reason for health care-related problems in a multicultural society where there is not a lot of diversity among healthcare providers—because when clashes and misunderstandings stem from different scripts, counterproductive illness behaviors may result.

TWO CLEAR EXAMPLES OF ILLNESS AND CULTURALLY SHAPED MORALITY

Leprosy (Hansen's Disease): The Classic Case of Stigma

Let's begin with the medical facts, insofar as they are known. Leprosy, or Hansen's disease, is a chronic, communicable disease affecting the skin, eyes, internal organs, peripheral nerves, and mucous membranes. The disease has been around for thousands of years, affecting every continent and ancient civilizations in China, India, and Egypt (World Health Organization, accessed at www.who.int/lep/leprosy). It is caused by two types of bacteria, *Mycobacterium leprae* and in some cases *Mycobacterium lepromatosis*, with genetic susceptibility possibly involved. Despite its time-worn reputation, leprosy is only mildly communicable; long-term contact (10–15 years) is necessary, and there is a long incubation period once infected. Treatment was not available until the 1940s, and the current multidrug therapy now cures the disease—resulting in a dramatic drop in prevalence to around 225,000 total cases (ibid.), from 10–12 million in the 1980s.

On its face, then, it's just a disease, like any other. Yet over the course of history it has become the most terribly stigmatizing of diseases, so much so that the generic term *leper* now refers to people who are shunned for many reasons.

Why? Because of the disfiguring physical symptoms, leprosy was and is still viewed with a kind of fear and abhorrence, leading to the historical association between leprosy victims and outcasts, and associations between that complex symbolic connection and divine punishment, or evil, or more generally, pollution. When a group of people is associated with pollution—as we will see with HIV/AIDS as well—other people don't want to

---

BOX 5-2 A Brief History of Leprosy

- A description of a disease that appears to be leprosy is recorded in an Egyptian papyrus document dated approximately 1550 BCE.
- Descriptions in India from about 600 BCE refer to a disease that resembles leprosy.
- In ancient Greece, leprosy is reported when the army of Alexander the Great returns from India; subsequently, it is also recorded in Rome in 62 BCE, coinciding with the return of Pompey's troops from Asia Minor.
- Throughout the intervening years, in many countries, leprosy was feared as a divine punishment, a curse, or a hereditary disease, and its victims shunned.
- In 1873, Norwegian doctor Gerhard Henrik Armauer Hansen first identified the bacteria that causes leprosy under a microscope (*Mycobacterium leprae*), showing it to be a disease like any other.
- An early treatment was to inject patients with the oil of the chaulmoogra nut—a painful treatment, though some success was reported.
- In 1941, a sulfone drug called "promin" was introduced. Its use required many painful injections, though it did successfully treat the disease.
- Dapsone pills were introduced in the 1950s. They were also successful, but the bacteria developed a resistance, reducing the effectiveness of the treatment.
- In the 1970s, a multidrug treatment that combined dapsone, rifampicin, and clofazimine was developed.
- Multidrug treatment therapy was recommended by the World Health Organization in 1981 and remains the current standard of treatment, though efforts continue to develop a vaccine.

Source: Adapted from Stanford University information site, www.stanford.edu/group/parasites/ParaSites2005/Leprosy/history.htm

---

have contact for fear of contamination. Leprosy has also been viewed as a sexually transmitted disease and as a consequence of witchcraft (Rafferty 2005; Scott 2000; Gilman 1999) and even as evidence that the victim is a witch. In Japan, the Shinto religion used the same word for leprosy and sin (Browne 1985). Until recently, there was no cure.

Consider a few examples of what happens to leprosy victims:

- In Nepal, and elsewhere in South Asia, victims often are divorced by their spouses, lose connection to their families, lose their jobs, and may be denied access to education. The impact is worse for women, whose role in their family may suffer (Rafferty 2005).
- In 1939, the Motor Vehicles Act in India forbade the granting of driver's licenses to leprosy victims, and until recently, the Indian Christian, Muslim, and Hindu marriage acts included leprosy as grounds for divorce (Bennett et al. 2008; Brown 2006).
- Leprosy victims were traditionally quarantined in isolated leper colonies, often with few resources and poor conditions. Well-known movies such as *Motorcycle Diaries* (2004) and *Papillon* (1973) have portrayed such colonies.

There may be other forces at work in the stigmatization of leprosy victims as well. Nancy Waxler (1998/1981) compares the experience of leprosy victims in several societies, concluding that the degree of stigma varies, and that both sociocultural and economic factors may be responsible. While the stigma, as noted earlier, is very strong in India, it is viewed somewhat differently, for example, among the Hausa in northern Nigeria. For the Hausa, leprosy is said to be caused by gluttony, swearing falsely by the Koran, or washing in the water a leprosy patient has used. Various treatments are practiced, including scraping or burning the skin. However, according to Waxler, it is viewed as just one disease among many. More telling, in Hawaii the severe reaction and quarantining of people with leprosy coincided with a rapid increase in Chinese immigration (to work on the plantations) during the mid and late 19th century. Due to racism and animosity (possibly economic) directed towards the Chinese by Americans in Hawaii, the Chinese likely became a scapegoat, and leprosy was the tool for its manifestation. Waxler adds that a leprosy patient

must *learn* to be a leper, a process in which people diagnosed with leprosy conform to the culturally shaped sick role for leprosy victims, stigmatizing themselves, and removing themselves from their homes, families, and communities.

HIV/AIDS: THE NEW LEPROSY

Now we come to the most stigmatized disease of modern times, known as acquired immune deficiency or AIDS. More properly, it is designated as HIV/AIDS because the immune deficiency is caused by the HIV virus. Infection by the HIV virus occurs via the following four basic channels:

1. As a sexually transmitted disease, through the exchange of body fluids during unprotected sex.
2. Through other exchanges of blood and body fluids that occur during the sharing of injection drug equipment and unsterilized needles, (including those used for tattoos).
3. Perinatal transmission—from mother to child during pregnancy, childbirth, or through breastfeeding.
4. Through the transfusion of contaminated blood.

Once infected, there is an incubation period of up to 10 years, and the virus then begins to destroy white blood cells called lymphocytes, progressively destroying the body's ability to fight disease. With little or no immunity, AIDS victims then suffer a host of other infectious diseases and cancers. Treatment involves various combinations of antiretroviral drugs, which slow down the replication of the virus but do not kill it. Perinatal transmission (mother to infant) can be blocked through the use of antiretroviral drugs such as azidothymidine (AZT).

HIV/AIDS AND STIGMA

On its face, HIV/AIDS is just a disease, like any other. Yet it emerged as a deeply stigmatized disease, right from its first appearance. As with leprosy, we are faced with the question, *why*? To a degree even greater than leprosy, HIV/AIDS hits very basic cultural, social, and political issues and seems to exert its impact along the

BOX 5-3 A Brief History of the HIV/AIDS Pandemic

- Several arguments have been made that the HIV virus originated in chimpanzees and may have infected humans as early as 1930 or earlier in what is now Zaire.
- Whatever its origins, the first AIDS symptoms were identified in the late 1970s among gay men. In 1981, the Centers for Disease Control and Prevention (CDC) began to report consistent symptoms among this population, a number of whom died.
- In 1982, CDC linked the disease to blood, and coined the terms *acquired immune deficiency syndrome* and *AIDS*.
- During 1983 and 1984, the HIV virus was discovered in France (at the Pasteur Institute) and by U.S. scientist Robert Gallo. There were already several thousand known deaths by this time. The first HIV antibody test was approved in 1985—the beginning of blood product testing.
- In 1986, Surgeon General Everett Koop published an important report on AIDS and called for sex education. By that time more than 16,000 deaths had occurred. AIDS became a national scare and received wide publicity. People who were infected or even at risk were shunned. Borders were closed to HIV-infected immigrants and travelers, and multiple problems surfaced with respect to discrimination and insurance (see, for example, the movie, *Philadelphia*, with Tom Hanks). By this time it was also clear that other populations were highly vulnerable, including injecting drug users.
- The first antiretroviral AIDS drugs (azidothymidine, zidovudine—generally referred to as AZT), were developed in 1987. After years of silence on the subject, then-U.S. President Ronald Reagan made his first speech concerning AIDS, and discrimination against federal employees with AIDS was prohibited in 1988.
- The Ryan White case in late 1980s brought national attention to the impact of discrimination and stigma. Ryan White was a young boy who had hemophilia and became infected with HIV through blood transfusions. Nevertheless, there was a public attempt to prevent him from attending middle school, and the controversy led him to become an activist against discrimination. Though he died in 1990, he remained a symbol of stigma issues surrounding HIV/AIDS. Later that year, Congress passed the Ryan White Care Act, which remains a major funding vehicle for a range of HIV/AIDS health and support services.
- Around that same time, a number of famous individuals in the U.S. and elsewhere died or were infected by HIV, including NBA star Magic Johnson. By the early 1990s, more than 10 million were infected worldwide.
- Following the success of azidothymidine, new antiretroviral drugs were developed and tested in the 1990s, and funding increased for prevention programs in the United States and globally. By 1995, annual known deaths in the United States alone approached 50,000. But with the introduction of more antiretroviral drugs and the development of multidrug (cocktail) therapies (highly active antiretroviral therapy or HAART), the mortality rate from AIDS began to drop after 1996 in locations where they were available. However, such treatments are expensive and have very limited availability in poor countries, bifurcating the consequences of the disease. By the late 1990s, the worldwide death toll approached 7 million, with more than 22 million infected. Sub-Saharan Africa and Thailand/Southeast Asia were among the hardest hit at that time. In the United States, AIDS moved from its original focus among gay men to other vulnerable populations—including women of color in high-poverty urban settings.
- The new millennium saw such developments as the Global Fund, changes in availability of drugs, etc., as well as the catastrophic consequences of AIDS in Sub-Saharan Africa and new areas of spread, including India, Russia, Eastern Europe, and China. New prevention options, including microbicides and rapid HIV testing methods, were introduced.
- In 2003, the Bush administration in the United States implemented a global effort called PEPFAR (President's Emergency Plan for AIDS Relief), targeting selected countries—most in Africa, but also China, Russia, Haiti, and others.
- Infection with HIV continues: In 2008, 2.7 million people were newly infected with HIV, and 2 million men, women, and children lost their lives. As of 2010, more than 34 million people around the world were living with HIV.

cracks and fissures in societies, among people who are most vulnerable.

HIV/AIDS intersects with very basic cultural territory, including:

- Gender relations (power)
- Gender roles (male, female, bisexual, transgender—the number of sexual partners accepted as normative)

FIGURE 5-1 HIV/AIDS Rally

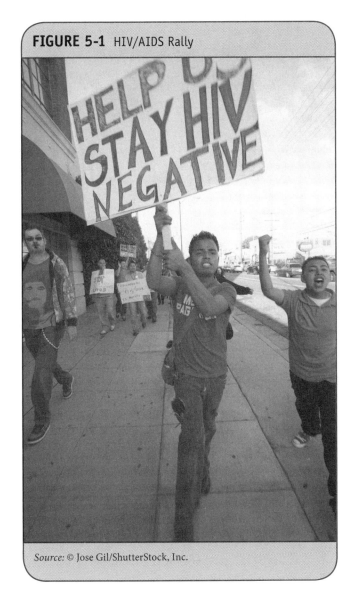

Source: © Jose Gil/ShutterStock, Inc.

- Sexuality and gender—definitions of appropriate/inappropriate sexuality and gender-related behavior
- Social stratification—hierarchies of wealth, power, and resources
- Family honor and shame

HIV infection is at first unseen and lies dormant, so it cannot always be identified. It therefore falls into line with ethnomedical systems that include supernatural and other-worldly forces as causal.

HIV/AIDS has also intersected with charged political issues. One of these issues concerns global ineq-

uity. The disease and virus were first discovered and gained prominence in Western developed countries, yet its origins have been tied to Africa. The association between Africa and HIV/AIDS carries with it an undertone of stigma, portraying Africa from the standpoint of Western countries as the other, as different—as the alien source. AIDS treatments were also developed in the West; they are expensive, require a health infrastructure, and have largely remained proprietary for the corporations that developed them, even though the disease has had its most severe impact in sub-Saharan Africa. This powerful juxtaposition has brought postcolonial politics into the mix, with some reactions against what are perceived as neocolonialist policies and attitudes. Perhaps the most well-known reaction of this kind was the resistance by South African President Thabo Mbeki and his health minister to accept the HIV virus as causal, and in turn to prohibit the distribution of antiretroviral drugs in public state hospitals.

HIV/AIDS disproportionally struck marginalized and disempowered communities. As a result, members of these communities have often viewed the prevalence of the disease as resulting from neglect, or even conspiracy.

It has been easy to blame HIV/AIDS on moral failure, because individual behavior is involved. The following have been implicated:

- Promiscuity and its meanings, whether same-sex or heterosexual
- Prostitution and its meanings—although *prostitution* is a complex and loaded term, applied at times to relationships of sex for resources (food, money, shelter) that don't always conform to the sex-market stereotype
- Intravenous drug use and drug addiction
- Motherhood and transmission to children

As Paul Farmer and Arthur Kleinman wrote, "AIDS has offered a new idiom for old gripes. We have used it to blame others: gay men, drug addicts, inner-city ethnics, Haitians, Africans. And we in the United States have, in turn, been accused of spreading and even creating the virus that causes AIDS" (1989: 137).

Yet there are social circumstances and poverty in both the developed and developing world that create conditions of high risk for infection with HIV. These conditions call into question easy moral judgments about a range of behaviors. When a woman must find any source of income to support children or a family and there are no options, the morality of exchanging sex for resources is complex. It is even more complex when, for example, this is compounded by a general lack of economic options for women, or rapid economic development that undercuts income-generating activity in rural villages necessitating migration to crowded urban areas, or when inner-city urban areas are isolated (through historical patterns of segregation and deindustrialization) from reasonable sources of income, and when globalized economic activity requires migration to find work, separating family members for long periods of time. Even a brief look at some of these circumstances raises the question: *Are there not moral failures in many of these circumstances themselves?*

STIGMA, METAPHOR, AND THE INSIGHTS OF SUSAN SONTAG

Susan Sontag (1933–2004) was an American writer, literary critic, social critic, and political and human rights activist who wrote two major, related works concerning illness and stigma—*Illness as Metaphor* (1978, on cancer) and *AIDS and Its Metaphors* (1988). In the latter work, she refers to the famous sociologist Erving Goffman's description of the effect of stigma as a spoiled identity. Thinking about her experience with cancer, Sontag framed her argument this way: "The metaphoric trappings that deform experience of having cancer have very real consequences: they inhibit people from seeking treatment early enough, or from making a greater effort to get competent treatment" (1978, 14). It is these stigma-creating metaphors and myths that actually kill. Her goal was to help people "regard cancer as if it were just a disease—a very serious one, but just a disease. Not a curse, not a punishment, not an embarrassment. Without 'meaning'" (1978, 102). Given all that we have covered so far in this book, the last comment is especially profound—in order to free cancer from stigma, she felt that she had to deprive it of meaning. Her follow-up work on HIV/AIDS and stigma shared a similar purpose. And in both books, she focused her attention on the role

BOX 5-4 What is a Metaphor?

Metaphor: A figure of speech in which one or more qualities of an object or idea are expressed through the use of an otherwise unrelated term. It is a significant means by which meaning is communicated through language and symbol. For example:

"Love is a rose"

"He was drowning in paperwork."

"Lately it has been a bull market."

of metaphor in public language as a key mechanism through which meaning is disseminated (and stigma created).

One form of metaphor highlighted by Sontag is what she calls the "military metaphor"—the use of military language and imagery to characterize all aspects of a disease, including HIV/AIDS.

> Military metaphors have more and more come to infuse all aspects of the medical situation. Disease is seen (and spoken of) as an invasion of alien organisms, to which the body responds by its own military operations, such as the mobilizing of immunological defenses,' and medicine is 'aggressive' as in the language of most chemotherapies. (Sontag 1988, 9)

While that may be relatively harmless, "Military metaphors contribute to the stigmatizing of certain illnesses and, by extension, of those who are ill." Illness victims then become the aliens, the invaders in our midst (Sontag 1988, 11).

For HIV/AIDS, two metaphors have been especially powerful, according to Sontag, representing the disease as both an invasion and as pollution. HIV/AIDS is viewed as exposing an identity (among those who are victims), which is a polluted or contaminated one (Sontag 1988, 25). The population groups who are at high risk and already stigmatized are thus "exposed" by HIV/AIDS. The pollution metaphor, says Sontag, has contributed to the construction of those afflicted with HIV/AIDS in a

FIGURE 5-2 Our Immune System is Like an Army

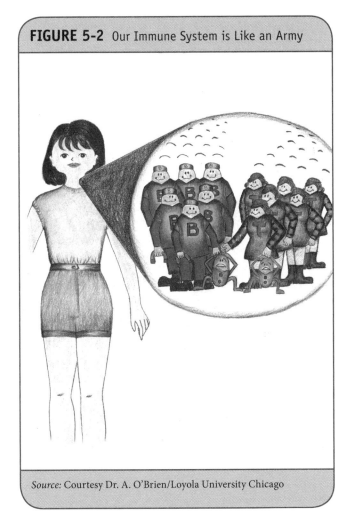

Source: Courtesy Dr. A. O'Brien/Loyola University Chicago

very different way than other diseases. It is not just those who are sick, but also those who are infected but have no symptoms—both are lumped together in discussions and statistics about HIV/AIDS.

The most powerful HIV/AIDS metaphor is said to be *plague*. "Plagues are inevitably regarded as judgments on society . . . and the metaphoric inflation of AIDS into such a judgment also accustoms people to the inevitability of global spread. . . . This is a traditional use of sexually transmitted diseases: to be described as punishments, not just of individuals but of a group" (Sontag 1988, 54). A plague is seen as a consequence of rejecting certain moral values—sexual values, behavioral values, religious values—and in that sense a form of pollution, easing the way to victim blaming. Particularly in the early stages of the pandemic, HIV/AIDS was portrayed in this way, as a kind of revenge of nature or divine

punishment. Victims became generalized as threats to society. "Epidemics of particularly dreaded illnesses always provoke an outcry against leniency or tolerance . . . now identified as laxity, weakness, disorder, corruption, unhealthiness" (Sontag 1988, 56–57).

Farmer and Kleinman echoed these insights about the public stigmatization of HIV/AIDS through metaphor:

> All illnesses are metaphors. They absorb and radiate the personalities and social conditions of those who experience symptoms and treatments. Only a few illnesses, however, carry such cultural salience they become icons of the times. Like tuberculosis in *fin de siecle* Europe, like cancer in the first half of the American century, and like leprosy from Leviticus to the present, AIDS speaks of the menace and losses of the times. It marks the sick person, encasing the afflicted in an exoskeleton of peculiarly powerful meanings: the terror of a lingering and untimely death, the panic of contagion, the guilt of "self-earned" illness. (1989: 137)

THE "OTHERING FUNCTION" OF CULTURE AND STIGMA

In a broader sense, the issue of stigma and the intersection of culture, morals and illness brings us to another social function of culture—we can call it the "othering function." The tendency for culture to provide a general coherence associated with a society or group means that the features of that coherent life pattern become integrated in, and valued as, the identity of people within that group: Saying, "We are *x*, we believe *y*, we do *z* (and this is good)," are all part of the same phenomenon. In fact, the name some cultural groups give to themselves, like the term *Dine* for Navajo peoples, actually means "the people." There is a flip side. When a group of people assert an identity, a sense of who they are, they are also creating a sense of difference—who they are *not*. People outside the group, who do not assert the same identity but other identities, which may entail other thoughts, beliefs and actions, are then by definition *the other*, as if saying, "We are the people. They are not."

And if there is a value attached to identity in a group, then there may be a concomitant and negative value judgment made about those who are viewed as *the other*. The oppositional characteristics of us and the other can be seen in numerous relational terms:

Our country/not from our country or foreigner
Our tribe/not in our tribe
Decent folk/not decent folk
With us/against us
Friends/enemies
Citizen/alien
Pure/polluted
Upstanding/decadent

There is also an element of fear connected with the other, the alien (think of all the 1950s movies about hostile invading aliens!), an existential fear that the alien somehow threatens social and cultural equilibrium. This is true whether the alien is an enemy of some kind or from a subgroup with a stigmatized illness. Thus stigma becomes a motive to suppress or deny the others, who

TABLE 5-1 Culture and Stigma		
Health problem	**Cause**	**Kind of person (other)**
Leprosy	Divine punishment	A bad person deserving of punishment
HIV/AIDS	Sexually loose morals	A promiscuous person
Cirrhosis of the liver	Addiction to alcohol or drugs	A weak person

are perceived to be a threat to the social whole. Taking it one step further, when illness stigma is woven within the structure of society, those who are stigmatized are often marginalized—cut off from the system of supports that contribute to prevention and healing. Marginalization amplifies health risk, resulting in an unnecessary and negative trajectory of illness.

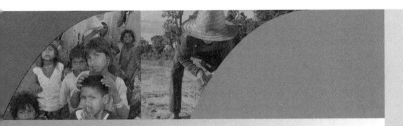

QUESTIONS

1. What other diseases/illnesses can you think of that are stigmatized? Why?

2. When do you think it is fair to point to individuals as at fault in terms of disease? When do you think it is fair to point to larger forces—at the societal level—as at fault?

3. Why do you think certain diseases are viewed as powerful moral threats, even greater than the actual impact of the disease? What seems to be at stake?

REFERENCES

Bennett, B.H., D.L Parker, and M. Robson. 2008. "Leprosy: Steps along the Journey of Eradication." *Public Health Reports* 123 (2): 198–205.

Brown, W. 2006. "Can Social Marketing Approaches Change Community Attitudes towards Leprosy?" *Leprosy Review* 77: 89–98.

Browne, S.G. 1985. "The History of Leprosy." In *Leprosy*, edited by R.C. Hastings. Edinburgh, Scotland and New York: Churchill Livingstone.

Chavez, L.R., F.A. Hubbell, and S.A. Mishra. 1999. "Ethnography and Breast Cancer Control among Latinas and Anglo Women in Southern California." In *Anthropology in Public Health*, edited by R.A. Hahn, 117–141. Oxford, England: Oxford University Press.

Collins, D., M.M. Villagran, and L. Sparks. 2008. "Crossing Borders, Crossing Cultures: Barriers to Communication about Cancer Prevention and Treatment Along the U.S.–Mexico Border." *Patient Education and Counseling* 71: 333–339.

Dumont, L. 1980. *Homo Hierarchicus: The Caste System and Its Implications.* Complete revised English ed. (first published in French, 1966). Chicago: University of Chicago Press.

Dumont, L. 1986. *Essays on Individualism: Modern Ideology in Anthropological Perspective.* Chicago: University of Chicago Press.

Edberg, M. 2007. *Essentials of Health Behavior: Social and Behavioral Theory in Public Health.* Boston: Jones and Bartlett.

Farmer, P., and A. Kleinman. 1989. "AIDS as Human Suffering." *Daedalus* 118 (2): 135–161.

Foucault, M. 1975. *The Birth of the Clinic: An Archaeology of Medical Perception.* Translated by A.M. Sheridan Smith. New York: Vintage/Random House.

Foucault, M. 1979. *Discipline and Punish: The Birth of the Prison.* Translated by Alan Sheridan. New York: Vintage/Random House.

Foucault, M., and C. Gordon, ed. 1980. *Power/Knowledge: Selected Interviews & Other Writings, 1972–1977.* Translated by C. Gordon, L. Marshall, J. Mepham, and K. Soper. New York: Pantheon Books.

France, A. 1894. *The Red Lily (Le Lys Rouge)* (trans. Winifred Stephens, 1921)—Punainen lilja (suom. Huvi Vuorinen, 1927).

Gilman, S.L. 1999. "Disease and Stigma." *Lancet* 354: SIV15.

Goffman, E. 1963. *Stigma: Notes on the Management of a Spoiled Identity.* New York: Simon & Schuster.

Kleinman, A. 1988. *The Illness Narratives: Suffering, Healing, and the Human Condition.* New York: Basic Books.

Kleinman, A., V. Das, and M. Lock, eds. 1997. *Social Suffering.* Berkeley: University of California Press.

Mshana, G., M.L. Plummer, J. Wamoyi, Z.S. Shigongo, D.A. Ross, D. Wight. 2006. "'She was Bewitched and Caught an Illness Similar to AIDS:' AIDS and Sexually Transmitted Infection Causation Beliefs in Rural Northern Tanzania." *Culture, Health & Sexuality* 8(1): 45–58.

Rafferty, J. 2005. "Curing the Stigma of Leprosy." *Leprosy Review* 76: 119–126.

Scott, J. 2000. "The Psychosocial Needs of Leprosy Patients." *Leprosy Review* 71: 486–491.

Singer, M. 2008. *Drugging the Poor: Legal and Illegal Drugs and Social Inequality.* Long Grove IL: Waveland Press.

Sontag, S. 1978. *Illness as Metaphor.* New York: Farrar, Straus & Giroux.

Sontag, S. 1988. *AIDS and Its Metaphors.* New York: Farrar, Straus & Giroux.

Thomas, F. 2007. "'Our Families are Killing Us:' HIV/AIDS, Witchcraft and Social Tensions in the Caprivi Region, Namibia." *Anthropology and Medicine* 14 (3): 279–291.

Waxler, N. 1998 (originally 1981). "Learning to Be a Leper: A Case Study in the Social Construction of Illness." In *Understanding and Applying Medical Anthropology*, edited by P. Brown, pp. 147–157. Mountain View, CA: Mayfield Publishing.

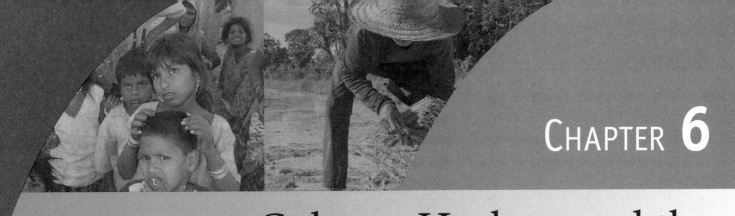

CHAPTER 6

Culture, Healers, and the Institutions of Health

"A bodily disease, which we look upon as whole and entire within itself, may, after all, may be but a symptom of some ailment in the spiritual part."

—Nathaniel Hawthorne, *The Scarlet Letter* (1850)

Following the logic of our discussion so far, let's move forward from considerations of health belief/knowledge systems and their potential moral dimensions to the next step in the process—healing. Once someone is identified as being ill, and the cause is ascertained, what does one do about it? Answering this question opens the door to a truly broad panorama of healers and healing practices across cultures. And because healers perform an essential cultural role in all societies, we must also consider healers in terms of the social institutions of healing.

THE SOCIAL INSTITUTIONS OF HEALING

This may be restating the obvious, but healers are not just anybody. While families and relatives play a role in healing, and may indeed be the first source of help, inevitably, people turn to one or more types of healers who are recognized as such and who operate within the ethnomedical systems and health provider structures prevalent in that society. This is not a random affair, or people would not know who to turn to or why. Healers are therefore embedded in a cultural process and at least some institutionalized practice or system so that individuals who are ill can make a decision about their treatment. In any society, this system in its entirety includes:

- The recognized typology of healers in society, whether these are *curanderos*, shamans, midwives, doctors, emergency medical technicians, physical

FIGURE 6-1 Connecting Illness and Cause to Healer and Treatment

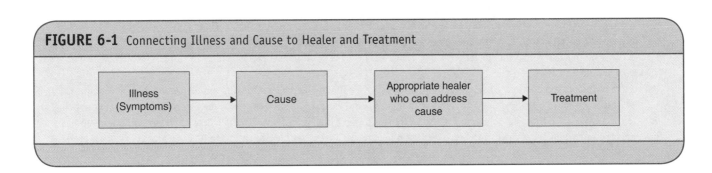

therapists, diviners, psychologists, or chiropractors; and the division of labor for these healers—for example, where some might be generalists and others specialists

- The physical sites of healing, whether hospitals, doctors offices, sweat lodges, or sacred spaces
- Rules/practices for regulating healers—who can be a healer, what are the boundaries of their practice, and how treatment success is evaluated
- Protocols for training healers—anything from apprenticeships to formal training and licensing
- A system of compensation through which the production of health is rewarded—whether this is in cosmic credits, barter, private payment, or via managed care
- In some societies, a social hierarchy of healers, in which some types of healers have more status, prestige, or power than others
- In some societies, organized groups of healers—for example, medical associations or healer's guilds.

TYPES OF HEALERS AND RITUALS OF HEALING

Across cultures, healing is practiced in an organized, ritualized form—healing ceremonies, divination, appointments, and so on. As such, all healing involves ritual and theater to a certain extent (e.g., uniforms such as white coats, chanting, aromas, the presence and participation of other community members, the use of implements and healing tools). Healing can therefore be thought of as a collective act. This is true whether the society is oriented to Western biomedicine or not. If you step outside your cultural box and take a look at biomedical practitioners, what occurs in a healing situation is neither pure technology nor pure science.

In a Western or biomedical ethnomedical system, what are the healers and their roles? In the following list, for example, what is the healing task of each of these healers?

- Doctors/general practitioners
- Surgeons

BOX 6-1 Legitimizing Healers

How do you know the healer you go to is legitimate and knows what he/she should know? Here are two examples:
- If you go to a medical doctor, what can you expect them to have done in terms of training? Most likely, they should have completed medical school and a residency or internship, passed the state licensing examination in order to have a license to practice, and possibly be board certified in a specialty or subspecialty.
- If you go to a shaman, what can you expect them to have done in terms of training? It varies, but in general, the shaman should have undergone an extensive apprenticeship to learn the practice, he or she should have evidence of a spiritual gift, either by lineage or through an experience, and he or she should have referrals or community affirmation of his or her effectiveness.

In Chapter 1, Laura Smith clearly doubted the legitimacy of the healer she went to, at first. As she climbed the stairs from the already-unconventional storefront entry, she scanned the scenario and felt unsettled because . . .
- The healer did not wear a white coat, so he did not look like a doctor.
- The room had none of the usual tools of the trade—stethoscope, blood pressure cuff, syringes, or sanitary wipes.
- There was no certification on the wall—no evidence of medical school or a license.
- The tools he did use (e.g., the dowel with its ornament, herbs, and aromatic candles) did not look anything like what a doctor should be using.

And so, he must not be a doctor, and what he is doing doesn't have anything to do with curing me, Laura must have thought.

Yet she did stay for a little while. She did talk to him. She did take the herbs with her when she left. And she almost considered using them. Why? Maybe *something* that he said resonated at least a little, although that initial opening was more or less canceled out when she went to the biomedical clinic, where, so to speak, her faith in the healing process was restored.

- Anesthesiologists
- Plastic surgeons
- Counselors/psychotherapists
- Physical therapists
- Nurses
- Physician assistants
- Emergency medical technicians
- Biomedical researchers

For each of these healers, consider the following: What is usually required to become one? Is it hereditary? Is it a special talent (e.g., from the divine)? Is training required? Is a certificate or diploma required? What else?

In ethnomedical systems that are not biomedically based, there are many types of healers. For example:

- Among the Akan-speaking Bono people of Ghana (portrayed in the film *Healers of Ghana*, from Films for the Sciences and Humanities), there are two types of healers and healing practices. The first, manifested in the *Minokua* ceremony, involves possession by a priest during which the deities accessed under possession inform the priest about the cause of the illness and which plants/herbs to use as a remedy. The second is a witch catching ceremony performed by an *obosombrafoo* (Konadu 2008), who identifies the individual(s) who have used the energy force known as *bayie* for negative purposes (often glossed as witchcraft), causing someone to become ill. Both draw on a concept of *sunsun*, the spiritual side of human nature, and on the coexistence of the living and a liminal or spirit world that play a role in daily affairs.
- In Mexico, Central America, and Latin America, a primary category of traditional healer is called a *curandero* (or if female, a *curandera*). *Curanderos* are both spiritual healer and herbal healer, and they can have various specialties depending upon their *don* or gift from God. Examples include *yerberos/yerberas* who specialize in a deep knowledge of herbs, *sobadoros/sobadoras* who perform massage, *espiritualistos/espiritualistas* who serve as psychic mediums, and *parteras* who focus on midwifery (Tafur, Crowe, & Torres 2009). Com-

mon to *curanderos*, regardless of specialty, is an understanding that there are natural ailments for which various natural remedies are appropriate and supernatural ailments that require intervention in that realm (Trotter & Chavira 1997), the latter category including, for example, *susto* (loss of soul) and *mal de ojo* (evil eye). Cures typically employ prayers, amulets, and spiritual rituals, as well as herbs, counseling, and lifestyle recommendations, and are often done in a family or collective setting (Maduro 1983). At the highest level of practice, some *curanderos* are said to use mental

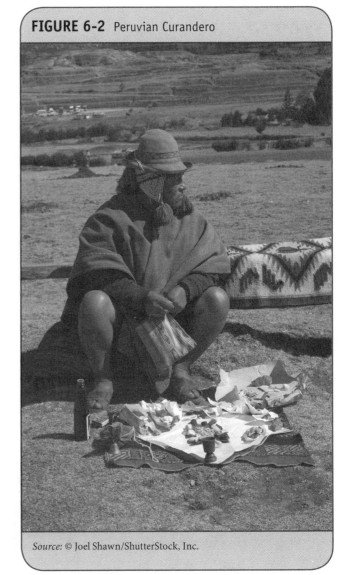

FIGURE 6-2 Peruvian Curandero

Source: © Joel Shawn/ShutterStock, Inc.

powers to harness energy towards the resolution of problems and illnesses.

- In the African-influenced, English-speaking cultural systems of the Caribbean (e.g., in Jamaica, Barbados, Trinidad and Tobago, St. Kitts, and others), a syncretic variant of West African spirit and witchcraft practices called "obeah" is common. A practitioner is an obeah man or obeah woman. Obeah is syncretic in that, like other Afro-Caribbean spiritual traditions, it combines African roots with European and Christian symbols (see Bilby & Handler 2004), and even Hindu symbols

(because of the long history of South Asians in the Caribbean). The term is used as a kind of catch-all to describe a broad collection of related practices and in that sense is less an organized religion than other African-influenced traditions of the region. Obeah practitioners engage in divination and the ritual manipulation of supernatural forces. While this can be used for negative ends, the most common and possibly original intent of obeah practitioners was to protect, to help ensure good fortune, to solve family or social problems, and to heal those who are ill (ibid.). Their work includes

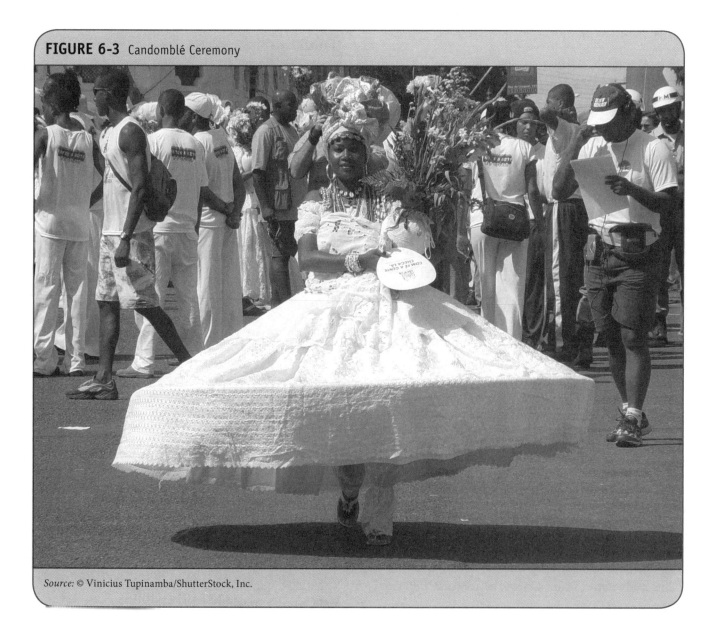

FIGURE 6-3 Candomblé Ceremony

Source: © Vinicius Tupinamba/ShutterStock, Inc.

the preparation of charms and amulets, herbal remedies, and divination rituals.

- *Candomblé* is practiced in Brazil—especially in the Bahia region (although it is also practiced in other parts of Latin America). It is a religion heavily influenced by Yoruba traditions from Nigeria, in which it is understood that every individual has personal spirits called *orixas*, who are intermediaries between them and the universe creator, Olorun (or Olodumare). There is also a spiritual force involved in healing called "*axe.*" Devotees of *Candomblé* increase their *axe* by daily devotional rites as well as possession ceremonies, in which drummers play rhythms that are specific to individual *orixas*, linked with specific dance steps, and induce possession. Healing rituals are conducted by priests, priestesses, and other healers, and healing occurs as part of collective rituals that spiritually empower both the person who is ill and others in the *Candomblé* community to help find solutions (DeLoach & Peterson 2010), as well as through the use of sacred herbs and plants (Voeks 1997).

- An important healer among the Hopi Indian people of the southwestern United States is the *Tuuhikya* (Grant 1982). Working within the partially naturalistic system of the Hopi Way, in which balance and harmony produce health, emotional balance is also viewed as necessary to maintain health—negative emotions such as anger, jealousy, envy, and hate can be associated with health problems. Like *curanderismo*, a distinction is made between natural and unnatural causes for illness, the latter which may include negative emotions/social actions, or even witchcraft (when the problem doesn't respond to other treatment). Diagnosis is an extended activity in which the healer attempts to understand the patient's history and circumstances, and some ritual is involved. Healing by the *Tuuhikya* may involve prayer, herbal preparations, rituals with feathers, smoke, crystals and other objects, as well as practical tools such as splints and bandages, and specific behaviors required of the patient (ibid.).

  Also for the Hopi, rainfall and other phenomena supporting community health and well-being come via the actions of supernatural beings called *kachinas*, who are spirits of the dead who return to intervene in nature on behalf of humans and are bearers of a life force (see Schaafsma 1994). During several ritual ceremonies, men wear *kachina* masks and costumes, and the spirit of these *kachinas* is said to enter the body of that person.

- In the Philippines, Brazil, parts of the Caribbean, and elsewhere, there are healers who perform what has been called "psychic surgery." This involves an apparent cut or incision made to a patient, the insertion of the psychic surgeon's hands inside the ill person, and the "removal" of diseased or polluting tissue, sometimes accompanied by what appears to be blood. Like other types of healing, psychic surgery involves a ritualized performance in a collective setting (Singer 1990).

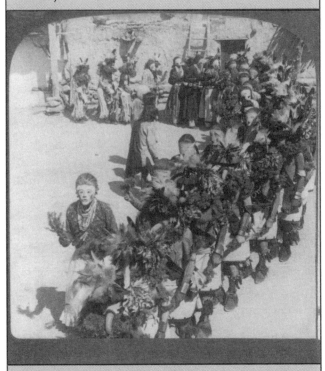

FIGURE 6-4 Kachina Dancer, Jemez Pueblo (New Mexico)

Source: Courtesy of Library of Congress Prints and Photographs Division, [Reproduction number: LC-USZ62-59803].

SHAMANS AND SHAMANIC HEALING PRACTICE: AN EXAMPLE OF HEALERS AND THEIR SOCIAL ROLE

A major cross-cultural category of non-biomedical healer is known as a "shaman." It has become something of a generic term for a broad range of spirit/herb healers, both men and women, and the term has arguably been misused in recent years in connection with a range of Western contemporary spiritual and healing practices sometimes referred to as "new age." Serious study of shamanism originated with reports of special healers among indigenous peoples in Siberia and has been broadened to include similar healers and practices around the globe. According to the Encyclopedia of Social and Cultural Anthropology, a shaman is a

> mediator between the human world and the world of spirits, between the living and the dead, and between animals and human society. Endowed with clairvoyance and assisted by helper spirits, a shaman fills many societal and religious roles, including those of soothsayer, therapist, and interpreter of dreams. He or she also plays an offensive and defensive role in the protection of his or her group against the aggressive actions of other shamans or displeased spirits. (Barnard & Spencer 1996, 504–508)

In other words, shamans are crossers of boundaries within the category systems of cultures. In other definitions (see Winkelman 2000, 2009; Eliade 1964), shamans are understood as utilizing altered states of consciousness (ASC) and collective healing rituals that draw from and stimulate biopsychological (neurological, emotional, consciousness-related) processes that can promote healing.

Because shamanic healing practices are so widespread and enduring, with evidence of healing effects, there has been growing interest in gaining a better understanding of what actually happens. In recent years, research efforts have sought to identify healing mechanisms that are harnessed in shamanic practices and rituals. Winkelman (2009; 2000), for example, has argued that shamanic healing and altered states of consciousness tap in to universal, physiological processes, including:

- Stimulation of serotonin neural pathways in the brain and the release of internally produced opioids. Serotonin (a neurotransmitter) and opioids are both associated with feelings of pleasure and well-being.
- Stimulation of the autonomic nervous system (ANS).
- Integrative activity in the brain, in which the three basic brain divisions (R-complex, limbic system, and neocortical structures—roughly corresponding to instincts/basic drives, emotions, and symbolic thought) are synchronized, producing a wide range of phenomena, including visions, metaphoric and prelinguistic thought, dream states, and a range of unconscious mental processes.
- Immune system stimulation.

Altered states of consciousness are often induced by extreme deprivation, rhythmic methods (drumming, chanting), physical exhaustion through dancing or other activity, auditory stimuli (music, bells), isolation, psychoactive drugs, and other methods. Cultures differ in the practices and technologies for inducing these states.

Like all healers, success for shamanic healers depends in part on the degree to which the healing practices are supported by community belief and, in many cases, participation. *To reiterate a message stated earlier, healing is a collective act.* As the anthropologist Claude Levi-Strauss wrote, "the efficacy of magic implies a belief in magic" (Levi-Strauss 1963, 168). It can be viewed as activity within a tautological belief system. There are three components of magic and healing: psychosomatic state of the shaman; healing experience (or not) of the client; and public/community participation.

Shamanic Healing and Performance. When a shaman engages in healing, it is important to energize the individual and collective psychological forces that contribute to healing, as described previously. This is done through a range of ritual performance practices. Here are a few examples:

- Music that involves chants and repeated rhythms, drumming.
- Ritual songs, invoking spiritual powers.
- The manipulation and use of symbolic objects— e.g., crosses, figurines, staffs, feathers, and altars

that include multiple symbols—to represent the forces that are brought to bear in healing.

- The entrance of the shaman (and possibly participants as well) into a trance (altered state of consciousness) state, during which the shaman is understood to be free of the confines of daily, earthbound experience and can travel in the world of the supernatural. This very important trance state may be generated in part through hallucinogenic substances like peyote, the San Pedro cactus, or iboga in Gabon and Zaire (Metzner 1998).

- A ritual sequence, through which spiritual power is invoked, attainment of a high energy point, and then the session is closed off with solutions and conclusions about the illness, its causes, and how to proceed. This may be followed by the prescription of a curative regimen and herbs.

Shamans as a Social Institution. Michael Brown, in an essay entitled, "Dark Side of the Shaman" (1989), writes about another aspect of the shaman as a healer. Because shamans are considered to have access to the supernatural, they play a social as well as a healing role. The two roles can be problematic. Brown describes a shaman he calls Yankush, among the Aguaruna of Peru.

BOX 6-2 Psychoactive Drugs and Shamanic Healers

- Among the Jivaro of Ecuador (see, for example, Harner 1984), shamans (and others) use a hallucinogenic drug called *natema*[a] in order to access and learn how to control spirits, who typically appear in the form of jaguars, birds, and snakes

- Shamans and others among the Yanamamo of the Amazon basin areas in Brazil use a drug called *ebene*[b] to access personal spirits (Peters 1998; Chagnon 1997). *Ebene* is actually curare, a poison that is also used on the tips of arrows. Ebene is snuffed up the nostrils, either by hand or through a bamboo tube.

---

a. Anthropologist Michael Harner took this drug and also reported seeing some of the same images, including the widely reported halo that appeared around the shaman.

b. The use of this kind of drug use is very different than what we often refer to as drug use here. It is highly ritualized, etc.

The Aguarana ethnomedical system is personalistic—thus serious illness is often said to be caused by sorcerers who put spirit darts into the bodies of their victims. If the darts aren't removed quickly, the victim will die. As discussed in Chapter 3, the sorcerer becomes a kind of criminal, and the act of making someone ill a crime motivated by bad intent. If a sorcerer is discovered, he is to be executed. However, sorcerers and shamans derive their power from the same source—one for evil, one for good. Sorcerers and shamans can both use spirit darts, but the work of a shaman is done in public, while that of a sorcerer is in secret. In the essay, Brown describes a precarious situation where Yankush is performing a healing. He is in a trance induced by the *ayahuasca* plant, and as the ceremony is conducted there are many comments from observers, some of which hint at the trouble Yankush could be in if his healing does not work—it will be assumed that the patient still has darts, and even that Yankush may have put them there (as if he were a sorcerer). As a shaman who works with the same powers as a sorcerer, Yankush is always under pressure to demonstrate that he is a healer. This requires him not only to be successful, but to agree to conduct healings that he may prefer to decline. In addition, Brown documents that to help insure his success, Yankush sometimes prescribed commercially available antibiotics or other medicines as well.

True to the predicament Brown described, Yankush was murdered in a sorcery-related vendetta 10 years after Brown wrote the essay.

NONBIOMEDICAL AND SPIRITUAL HEALERS IN WESTERN/DEVELOPED COUNTRIES

To make sure that the idea of traditional, non-biomedical and spiritual healers is not presented here as an exotic phenomenon, only found in non-Western countries, it is useful to be reflexive. Make no mistake, such healers have long been part of the social fabric in the United States as well as in Europe, from country medicine peddlers and spiritual mediums to more current faith healers and holistic health practitioners. Let's take a look at some of these practices and institutions.

The National Center for Complementary and Alternative Medicine. In the United States, the cultural

BOX 6-3 Was Jimi Hendrix a Shaman?

Jimi Hendrix was the iconic and gifted guitar player who changed the way the electric guitar was used in rock as well as jazz and other music genres. He died in 1970 under circumstances that are still unclear, related to a drug overdose. While he is known for his guitar wizardry and genius for using the electric guitar and recording technologies in creating an other-worldly spectrum of sound, to some, Jimi Hendrix was an unusual, theatrical performer who seemed to be in touch with deep, supernatural powers. His music, and performances, were often transfixing, and mesmerizing, and his entire body and soul seemed to be carried away to another plane as he played.

Perhaps the most well-known example is his startling performance at the Monterey Pop Festival in 1967, when he treated his guitar as a sacrificial object and burned it on stage, calling forth the flames as if calling forth its spirit. In another performance, at the famed Woodstock festival in 1969 and during the height of antiwar protests, he played an ethereal and emotional Star Spangled Banner to the depleted, exhausted morning audience, pulling and bending his guitar, scraping it across the microphone, and piercing the ringing patriotic melody with the sounds of exploding bombs and anguished cries, as if he were channeling the very souls of those killed in the warfare.

Was he a shaman?

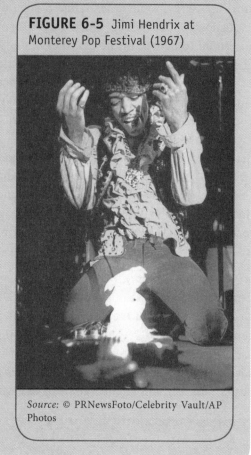

FIGURE 6-5 Jimi Hendrix at Monterey Pop Festival (1967)

Source: © PRNewsFoto/Celebrity Vault/AP Photos

opening brought on during the 1960s to non-Western philosophies and healing practices laid the foundation for serious examination and use of alternative medicine, including acupuncture and meditation, as well as a proliferation of natural food and health stores (now Internet sites) where a range of herbal remedies became available. Because so many claims have been made for these kinds of therapies, scrutiny has increased, and more have become the focus of scientific research. In 1998, the National Center for Complementary and Alternative Medicine (NCCAM) was founded, becoming one of the institutes and centers that make up the National Institutes of Health within the U.S. Department of Health and Human Services. NCCAM is the lead agency

for scientific research on complementary and alternative medicine, and its mission is to explore complementary and alternative healing practices in the context of rigorous science; train complementary and alternative medicine researchers; and disseminate authoritative information to the public and professionals. NCCAM sponsors and conducts research using scientific methods and advanced technologies to study complementary and alternative medicine (CAM)—understood as referring to the diverse medical and healthcare systems, practices, and products that are not currently considered to be part of conventional biomedicine. However, at this point NCCAM tends to focus on a relatively limited set of these alternative practices.

Pennsylvania Dutch Pow-Wowers. Among the various Pennsylvania Dutch groups in the United States (e.g., Amish, Mennonite) there is a folk-healing tradition that was for the most part hidden until interest began to grow in alternative health (Offner 1998). This tradition is called "pow-wowing" and has its origins in the pagan practices of the Druids in Europe (Offner 1998; Ravenwolf 1995), with the use of magic, mysticism, and spiritualism from ancient Wicca (white magic) practices of tribal Germany. Herbal remedies and potions are a part of the rural German tradition as well, and some practices were incorporated from interaction with American Indian peoples. The Pennsylvania Dutch healers take a cooperative perspective with respect to biomedical practitioners.

Pow-wowers are formally trained, and before training begins, they choose whether to practice as Christian faith healers or pagan/Wicca practitioners; both are viewed as drawing from the same energy (Offner 1998). However, the power to be a healer is considered to run in families, and is handed down in a ceremony called the "passing of power" (ibid.). The training takes several years and focuses on learning to harness one's own energy, the protocols for examining seven areas of the body that are said to reveal balances or imbalances of heat and energy, manipulation of energy flow, diagnostic procedures, and the use of chanting, charms, herbs, animal totems, and runes.

Acupuncturists. Rooted in Chinese medicine and its naturalistic ethnomedical roots (see Chapter 3), acupuncture has become one of the most widely used and now experimentally tested alternative healing approaches in the United States and the West in general. It is based on a complex system of states of being that are derived from the two general complementary forces of yin and yang (see Kaptchuk 2002), which are related to physical, spiritual, and emotional aspects of well-being. The underlying force that links these aspects of well-being together is *Qi* (pronounced "chee"). According to the theory behind acupuncture, there are 365 pressure points, located on 14 main channels (ibid.) throughout the body, that form a web of access to the sources of yin and yang throughout the body. An acupuncturist diagnoses the disharmony in these forces that is the cause of the health problem and then uses the insertion of nee-

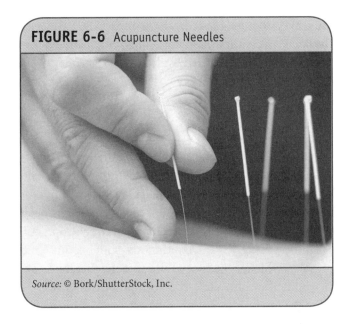

FIGURE 6-6 Acupuncture Needles

Source: © Bork/ShutterStock, Inc.

dles, along with pressure and sometimes heat, to move the Qi and restore harmony to the complex of forces in the body, which should then be reflected in better health. There have been some randomized and scientific studies of acupuncture, providing evidence that it is effective in reducing pain, reducing nausea following chemotherapy and during pregnancy, and even with other issues such as smoking cessation.

Acupuncturists can be found all over the Western world, in settings that range from storefronts and Chinese/herbal medicine stores to clinics/practices specializing in the therapy. In the United States, California was the first state to license acupuncture as a therapy, and as of 2002 (Kaptchuk 2002) 40 states and the District of Columbia had followed suit.

Chiropractors. Although chiropractic as a form of manipulative therapy is recognized and licensed in the United States, it is not generally well understood by most people and has a different history than biomedicine. Chiropractic shares roots with other similar therapies and spinal manipulation techniques practiced in Indonesia, Hawaii, Japan, China, India, Central Asia, Mexico, Nepal, Russia, and Norway. The Western roots of manipulation approaches have been traced back to Hippocrates and ancient Greece (around 400 BCE) and to other noted figures in the history of medicine (Pettman 2007). In the United States, the origins of modern chiropractic are linked to a magnetic healer named D.D. Palmer in the late 19th century (Homola 2006), who theorized that most diseases were caused by displaced vertebrae, or by "luxations" of other joints.

Palmer's central idea was that bodily functions are controlled by the flow of nerve vibrations from the brain to the spinal cord and then through openings in the vertebrae (ibid.). When one or more vertebrae move out of position, they are said to create pressure on or irritate spinal nerves (subluxation), which then causes malfunction, leading to health problems. This thesis has been disputed by biomedical researchers, but the chiropractic profession disagrees and continues to support this basic premise, which is the root of chiropractic therapy. Most chiropractors also view the chiropractic tradition as aligned with holistic health perspectives, linking health problems to the function of the body's systems as a whole, not just discrete organs or parts. There have been historical disputes as well between chiropractors and practitioners of other forms of physical and manipulative therapy (Pettman 2007).

Chiropractors can be found across the United States. Typically, they are trained in and use a range of spinal manipulation techniques, and sometimes use a handheld, spring-loaded metal device called an "activator," which is intended to tap vertebrae into alignment. There are several organizations for chiropractors, including the American Chiropractic Association and the International Chiropractic Association, as well as the Association of Chiropractic Colleges.

THE TRUTH OF HEALERS— BIOMEDICAL VS. TRADITIONAL

Assessing whether or not something works within the biomedical tradition is typically clear-cut. Either the inflammation is reduced or it isn't. Either the bacteria are eliminated or they aren't. Either the bone heals or it doesn't. The truth of biomedicine lies in the empirical evidence of its elimination of symptoms and/or of the cause—essentially, pathogens, or body malfunctions. That evidence is obtained through research using the scientific method, using data measuring symptoms as well as the presence of causal agents. The same standards are often applied as a measure of effectiveness

to non-biomedical traditions, though with reference to the causes that are part of a given ethnomedical system. However, there are important qualitative differences. As you now know, non-biomedical approaches often focus on causal factors larger than just the specific health problem at hand—for example, restoring balance, or addressing spiritual issues or social relationships. These are by nature harder to measure empirically and harder to link precisely to a specific set of symptoms.

There are also pragmatic issues to consider. If you think about a psychic surgeon as a healer, it may be empirically clear that the treatment of pulling out diseased tissue is not "true." That may not, in fact, be what the psychic surgeon is doing, and in that respect it is a hoax (Singer 1990). But the question remains—so what? What if the whole enterprise of psychic surgery is viewed as completely symbolic, as a cultural production, and that the cooperative belief system of both healer and patient itself contributes to curing? It is then possible to look at this problematic from another point of view, in which the empirical validity of the specific procedure is not the issue. According to Melvin Konner:

> All folk healing systems—and modern scientific medicine too—are based on the relationship between the healer and the victim of illness. The behavioral and psychological features of this relationship—such elements as authority, trust, shared beliefs, teaching, nurturance, and kindness—significantly, and sometimes dramatically, affect the course of illness, promoting healing, and preventing recurrence . . . Call it placebo if you like, but the human touch has a real and measurable effect. (2010, 113)

It doesn't necessarily matter, then, if the psychic surgery is empirically valid as a discrete procedure, because what it may be doing is contributing to a psychological state within the patient, and within the social support mechanisms of the patient, in which there is a shared belief that a cure is at hand. Of course, that in itself may not be enough to actually produce a cure. But it may help, especially if combined with other forms of therapy. So the question of truth takes on a different dimension.

Finally, go back to the placebo effect (described in Chapter 3). When empirical research demonstrates that a significant percentage of patients who are ill report improvement in symptoms after taking a placebo, is it actually a cure? Or should it be called a "curative agent?" What is the truth here?

DRAWING FROM MULTIPLE TRADITIONS

There have been numerous efforts in recent years to take the more holistic, psychological, and symbolic effects of traditional healing practices and combine this aspect with biomedical practice as a collaboration. Some of the most well-documented examples of such collaboration concern efforts to address HIV/AIDS in sub-Saharan Africa. There are at least three factors that have contributed to this trend: (1) the prevalence of indigenous healing and healers; (2) the difficulty in accessing biomedical doctors for much of the population; and (3) the expense and often limited accessibility to testing and antiretroviral therapy (drugs) for many people. So in several countries, a collaborative pattern has emerged, where indigenous healers work with biomedical practitioners in implementing prevention programs as well as in managing the complications resulting from HIV/AIDS. Traditional healers are in the community and available 24 hours a day. They are already respected for advice on well-being. Most reports also indicate that traditional healers are very supportive of collaboration and have already established patterns of referral to biomedical practitioners for emergency cases and other acute problems. In working with a biomedical practitioner, the traditional healer can focus on disseminating—and legitimizing—prevention information and on counseling individuals about risk behavior; accompanying individuals to testing or treatment; addressing the psychological trauma associated with the disease; helping (with herbal remedies) to treat such symptoms as sores; and generally looking after the well-being of the patient and his/her family. The biomedical practitioner's role is focused on diagnosis and the administration of specific treatments.

There are other examples as well.

Thai Traditional Medicine and Biomedicine. Although Thailand's health system is primarily modern biomedicine, in the 1970s there was a revival of Thai traditional medicine (TTM) following the WHO/UNICEF Alma Ata Declaration in 1978, urging member countries to increase primary care coverage using all available resources, including indigenous resources (Chokevivat and Chuthaputti 2005), and a general movement to integrate TTM into the national health system. TTM is based on practices and books handed down across generations, congruent with Thai culture and with Buddhism. "TTM uses various forms of practices to complement each other, i.e., medicine, pharmacy, massage, midwifery and maternal and child health care, Buddhist rites and meditation, as well as other rituals based on the belief in supernatural power or power of the universe" (ibid., 1–2). In some ways reflective of Ayurvedic medicine, TTM holds that there are four main elements (*tard*) in the body—earth, water, wind, and fire—and that in each person one of those elements (*tard-chao-ruan*) is dominant. This also varies by life cycle stage. Illness can be caused by supernatural power (including ancestors, spirits, etc.); the power of nature as manifested by imbalances in the four elements, hot/cold imbalances, or general imbalances in equilibrium; the power of the universe (sun, moon, stars); and *kimijati*—analogous to microorganisms or parasites in biomedicine.

An integrated diagnostic examination may include procedures common to biomedicine (pulse, heart rate, temperature), as well as an assessment of habits/practices that can cause imbalance, and an astrological examination. Treatments are generally holistic in relation to general well-being, as well as Thai massage, baths, herbal compresses, and other procedures.

As TTM gained currency in medical and health practitioner circles, units were created in the Thai Ministry of Health to organize and manage the practice of TTM, culminating in the recent creation in 2002 of the Department for the Development of Thai Traditional and Alternative Medicine within the ministry. A college for the study of TTM has been established, and graduates can take a licensing examination to become applied TTM practitioners. The Foundation for the Promotion of Thai Traditional Medicine, with other organizations, also revived and publishes the classic TTM textbook, called *Tumra Paetsart Sonkhrau.*

Integration of Hmong Shamans into Hospital Care in California. Following the large influx of Hmong refugees from Laos into California's Central Valley in the late 1970s and early 1980s, it became clear that there was a large gap between Hmong and biomedical health practices, sometimes resulting in disaster—as tragically described for epilepsy patient Lia Lee in Anne Fadiman's *The Spirit Catches You and You Fall Down* (see profile in Chapter 3). Adapting to the needs of Hmong patients, and in keeping with a general need for hospitals to understand the increasing diversity of patients, Mercy Hospital in Merced began to implement a training program to integrate Hmong shamans into the care system (Brown 2009) and to increase their familiarity with biomedicine in order to help allay some of the fears about surgery, blood transfusions, and other procedures that keep many in the Hmong community away from the hospital even when treatment is needed. Shamans who complete the training wear embroidered jackets and official badges and are granted the same kind of unrestricted access to patients accorded to members of the clergy.

They can perform *soul callings* and other protective and healing rituals, and (with hospital permission) can use gongs, finger bells, incense and other ritual tools. Biomedical doctors at Mercy Hospital became supportive of the integration policy after publicity surrounding the case of Lia Lee, and when they saw that treatment of Hmong patients was much more successful when combined with traditional shamanic practice. Furthermore, Hmong patients are much more likely to go for treatment if they know that a shaman will be there as well.

Indigenous Healers for High Risk Youth in Hawaii. Given the increasing push for culturally competent health care in the United States and the need for prevention as a means of reducing healthcare costs, there has been increasing interest in Hawaii to support the use of native Hawaiian healers as part of an integrated system of care (Bell et al. 2001). The Native Hawaiian Health Care Act of 1988 specifically called for support of such an effort. This may be especially important for Native Hawaiian youth who have had higher rates of morbidity and mortality related to a range of high-risk behaviors (e.g., substance abuse, sexual risk, violence), in part due to cultural marginalization and socioeconomic factors. Since adolescence as a developmental stage involves a

process of identity development, experience has often shown that greater cultural attachment and identity increases *resilience* and helps prevent higher risk behavior patterns. Indigenous Hawaiian healers (generally called "kahunas") are typically used for psychosocial problems or when a patient is told by a biomedical doctor that there is nothing wrong, even though he/she is experiencing symptoms (ibid.). Youth who are involved in high-risk behavior are more likely to have psychosocial issues. To link a culture-strengthening process with healing, organizations such as the Native Hawaiian Mental Health Research Development Program and the University of Hawaii's John A. Burns School of Medicine, the Hawaii Primary Care Association, and Papa Ola Lokahi (nonprofit) have been at the forefront, supporting the dissemination of knowledge about Native Hawaiian healing and increasing access to these services as a complement to biomedical practice.

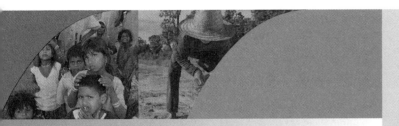

QUESTIONS

1. What signs and symbols could the healer have employed to make patients like Laura Smith more accepting of what he was trying to do?

2. Has anyone in your family ever given you something or done something that made you feel better when you were sick, even though it wasn't medical in the strict sense?

3. Given the increasing diversity of the U.S. population and your understanding of cross-cultural healing, can you think of a policy approach that might help the healthcare system be more effective in the future?

4. In your neighborhood or city, have you ever noticed any healthcare practitioners who are not biomedical? Have you ever made use of any of these practitioners?

5. Whether biomedical or not, are there any personal qualities or abilities that contribute to the effectiveness of a healer or health practitioner? Why are those qualities/capabilities helpful?

6. Have you ever been at an event, such as a religious event, concert, or a music or drumming performance in which you felt caught up or at one with the audience and musicians? What was that situation?

REFERENCES

Barnard, A., and J. Spencer. 1996. *Encyclopedia of Social and Cultural Anthropology.* London: Routledge.

Bell, C.K., D.A. Goebert, R.H. Miyamoto, E.S. Hishinuma, N.N. Andrade, R.C. Johnson, J.F. McDermott, Jr. 2001. "Sociocultural and Community Factors Influencing the Use of Native Hawaiian Healers and Healing Practices among Adolescents in Hawai'i." *Pacific Health Dialog* 8 (2): 249–259.

Bilby, K.M., and J.S. Handler. 2004. "Obeah: Healing and Protection in West African Slave Life." *The Journal of Caribbean History* 38 (2): 153–183.

Brown, M.F. 1989. "Dark Side of the Shaman." *Natural History* 11: 8–10.

Brown, P.L. 2009. "A Doctor for Disease, a Shaman for the Soul." *New York Times*, September 20. www.nytimes.com/2009/09/20/us/20shaman.html.

Chagnon, N.A. 1997. *Yanomamo: The Fierce People*, 5th ed. Austin, TX: Holt, Rinehart & Winston, Inc.

Chokevivat, V., and A. Chuthaputti A. 2005. "The Role of Thai Traditional Medicine in Health Promotion." Paper presented at the WHO 6th Global Conference on Health Promotion Policy and Partnership for Action: Addressing the Determinants of Health. Bangkok: Thailand, August 7–11.

DeLoach, C.D. and M. Petersen. 2010. "African Spiritual Methods of Healing: The Use of Candomble in Traumatic Response." *The Journal of Pan-African Studies* 3 (8): 40–65.

Eliade, M. 1964. *Shamanism: Archaic Techniques of Ecstasy.* New York: Pantheon Books.

Grant, R.E. 1982. "Tuuhikya: The Hopi Healer." *American Indian Quarterly* 6 (3/4): 291–304.

Harner, M.J. 1984. *The Jivaro: People of the Sacred Waterfalls.* Berkeley, CA: University of California Press. (First published in 1972 by the Natural History Press, then by Anchor Press/Doubleday in 1973).

Homola, S. 2006. "Chiropractic: History and Overview of Theories and Methods." *Clinical Orthopaedics and Related Research* 444: 236–242.

Kaptchuk, T.J. 2002. "Acupuncture: Theory, Efficacy and Practice." *Annals of Internal Medicine* 136: 374–383.

Konadu, K. 2008. "Medicine and Anthropology in Twentieth Century Africa: Akan Medicine and Encounters with (Medical) Anthropology." *African Studies Quarterly* 10 (2 and 3): 45–69.

Konner, M. 2010. "Transcendental Medication." In *Understanding and Applying Medical Anthropology*, 2nd ed., edited by P.J. Brown and R. Barrett. New York: McGraw-Hill.

Levi-Strauss, C. 1963. "The Sorcerer and His Magic." In *Structural Anthropology, Volume I*, edited by C. Levi-Strauss. New York: Basic Books.

Maduro, R. 1983. "*Curanderismo* and Latino Views of Disease and Curing." *The Western Journal of Medicine* 139: 868–874.

Metzner, R. 1998. "Hallucinogenic Drugs and Plants in Psychotherapy and Shamanism." *Journal of Psychoactive Drugs* 30 (4): 333–341.

Offner, J. 1998. "Pow-wowing: The Pennsylvania Dutch Way to Heal." *Journal of Holistic Nursing* 16: 479–486.

Peters, J.F. 1998. *Life among the Yanomami: The Story of Change among the Xilixana on the Mucajai River in Brazil.* Orchard Park, NY: Broadview Press.

Pettman, E. 2007. "A History of Manipulative Therapy." *The Journal of Manual and Manipulative Therapy* 15 (3): 165–174.

Ravenwolf, S. 1995. *Hexcraft: Dutch Country Pow-Wow Magick.* St. Paul, MN: Llewellyn.

Schaafsma, P., ed. 1994. *Kachinas in the Pueblo World.* Albuquerque, NM: University of New Mexico Press.

Singer, P. 1990. " 'Psychic Surgery:' Close Observation of a Popular Healing Practice." *Medical Anthropology Quarterly* 4 (4): 443–451.

Tafur, M.M., T.K. Crowe, and E. Torres. 2009. "A Review of *Curanderismo* and Healing Practices among Mexicans and Mexican-Americans." *Occupational Therapy International* 16 (1): 82–88.

Trotter, R.T. II, and J.A. Chavira. 1997. *Curanderismo: Mexican-American Folk Healing*, 2nd ed. Athens, GA: University of Georgia Press.

Voeks, R.A. 1997. *Sacred Leaves of Candomblé: African Magic, Medicine and Religion in Brazil.* Austin, TX: University of Texas Press.

Winkelman, M. 2000. *Shamanism: The Neural Ecology of Consciousness and Healing.* Westport, CT: Bergin & Garvey.

Winkelman, M. 2009. *Culture and Health: Applying Medical Anthropology.* San Francisco, CA: Jossey-Bass.

CHAPTER 7

Sociocultural Ecologies of Disease and Illness

"How society waits unform'd, and is for a while between things ended and things begun"

—Walt Whitman, from *Leaves of Grass* (1860)

So far, we have talked about peoples and cultures and their relationship to health beliefs and practices. We now have to take the discussion a step further. People and cultures, and the patterns of disease and illness that occur within cultural settings, also interact with various environments—physical, biological, political, and socioeconomic. That process of interaction can be thought of as an *ecology*, in the same way that any species interacts with an environment and is part of an ecology. In the case of people and culture, over time the ecology helps shape characteristics of the culture, and in turn those characteristics create constraints and boundaries for people within a culture.[1] Within specific ecologies, people and cultures adapt to the environments they are faced with—sometimes in ways that work out well, other times in ways that are more problematic. Sound complicated? Well, it is—but hopefully these relationships, and how they affect health, will be clarified as you go through the chapter.

---

[1] Culturally-generated action may also alter the external environment (physical, biological, political, socioeconomic), changing the nature of the interaction.

VULNERABILITY

A key concept in trying to understand how health is affected through interaction with different ecologies is the idea of *vulnerability*. To illustrate this, think of a hypothetical culture called the "Chalmy" (a completely arbitrary, made-up name). Let's say that Chalmy culture is closely tied to small farming. Right now, however, the Chalmy people are living in a physical setting where there are occasional droughts, resulting in a pattern of

---

BOX 7-1 **What Do We Mean by** *Ecology?*

- Concept originally from biology (that, in any case, is its metaphoric reference)
- Refers to a system of interactions between organisms and an environment
- Refers to the complex relationships between organisms in the system—e.g., niches, hierarchies, dependencies, interdependencies
- Assumes that, over time, the ecosystem is maintained (in a state of homeostasis, more or less) through the dependent interaction of members of the system—such that if the system is disrupted, an imbalance occurs and the system may malfunction (at least temporarily), but then correct itself or adjust.

living that involves a high vulnerability to the health problem of malnutrition. Now let's assume that Chalmy culture, evolved over centuries, places a high value on farming methods that are not as effective as could be against drought, in part because the land they lived on for a long time was not so prone to drought. The interaction between Chalmy culture and the current drought-prone environment will lead to even greater vulnerability to malnutrition for the society as a whole.

Now we will add another layer to the picture. A big reason that the Chalmy are living in a more difficult environment than in their past (leading to the mismatch between their farming methods and values and the actual environment) has to do with the broader political environment. Much of their traditional land, it turns out, is oil rich. So for decades, the Chalmy have been pushed off the best part of that land to areas where the weather is less predictable and sometimes very dry. The political system in the country where the Chalmy live is controlled primarily by people who are not Chalmy and who are seeking to profit from a global economy in which oil means big money, and where big money in turn allows the government to purchase technologies—including weapons. These technologies increase their power and make it that much harder for the Chalmy to challenge their situation. So their relationship with the physical environment is in part determined by their relationship to a broader political and economic environment, accentuating an ecology of vulnerability.

Now let's add yet one more layer, this time internal to Chalmy culture. Chalmy social structure involves a hierarchy based on clan or lineage, with the most privileged clan seen as direct descendants of the mythical founder of the Chalmy people, named Chalmeus. Even though the Chalmy people are now all living on and farming land that is not great, the Chalmeus clan gets the best of the land that they do have and has priority access to wells. So, internally, some Chalmy are more vulnerable to malnutrition than others.

What we have described here are layers of vulnerability, created by a specific sociocultural and political ecology. It doesn't *have to* be that way, but the combined layers of cultural and political relationships, interacting with a physical environment, have produced a situation in which:

- All Chalmy are more vulnerable to malnutrition than non-Chalmy
- Some Chalmy are even more vulnerable to malnutrition than other Chalmy

Can you see that the cultural connection to disease and illness, which will still include all the cultural components we talked about before in terms of ethnomedical system and healers, is affected by broader factors as well—that are also linked to culture? The key is that vulnerability is to some degree arbitrary, based on social, cultural, and political-economic configurations. The situation faced by the Chalmy is not a given—except, perhaps for their original location within a physical environment.

In more general terms, at the societal level, societies and communities are all exposed to pathogens and environmental risks. The degree to which these exposures have an impact on the society has to do with both the nature of the risk and the vulnerability of that society—which in turn has to do with the society's resources, capacities, and other characteristics. Some societies are therefore more vulnerable than others.

At the individual level, individuals within societies are all exposed to pathogens (bacteria, germs) and many individuals experience other kinds of physical challenges and problems. Exposure to pathogens alone is not sufficient for an individual to become ill. It depends upon how physically vulnerable that individual is—which is related to his or her level of nutrition, access to resources, access to health care, exposure to the stressors of poverty or other conditions, and so on. The existence of physical problems in itself is not sufficient for an individual to be incapacitated. Again, this depends upon similar kinds of vulnerabilities. Within societies, then, some individuals are more vulnerable than others. When groups of individuals within a society share a pattern of health vulnerability, we can think of it as a *trajectory*.

The question we need to examine is *why?* What factors cause differential vulnerabilities? The answer has to do with the complex interplay of physical, sociocultural, and political-economic layers that form a particular ecology of disease. Now we'll go through these ecological layers in more detail, beginning with physical environments and moving to sociocultural and political-economic environments—with the understanding that these layers overlap.

CULTURE, THE PHYSICAL ENVIRONMENT, AND DISEASE

Some patterns of vulnerability to disease are driven by the interaction between a society/cultural group and a physical environment. In a nutshell, this means that the beliefs, social organization, and living pattern of a particular culture are causing that culture to adapt well to a disease environment, not to adapt well, or even to exacerbate a disease or other health threat. A few examples should help clarify this.

A number of classic examples of disease vulnerability can be found in Jared Diamond's *Guns, Germs and Steel* (1999), focusing on variation in the histories of livestock domestication and how these culturally specific histories exposed the domesticators to pathogens that evolved into human diseases—for example, measles, tuberculosis, and smallpox originally from cattle and flu from pigs and ducks. Speaking about early (and continuing) farming practices that accelerate the spread of disease, such as the use of human/animal feces for fertilizer, Diamond writes:

> Irrigation agriculture and fish farming provide ideal living conditions for the snails carrying schistosomiasis and for flukes that burrow through our skin as we wade through the feces-laden water. Sedentary farmers become surrounded not only by

their feces but by disease-transmitting rodents, attracted by the farmers' stored food. The forest clearings made by African farmers also provide ideal breeding habitats for malaria-bearing mosquitos. (1999, 205)

In an example of positive adaptive practices, Peter Brown (2010) describes the interaction between cultural patterns and malaria in Sardinia, an island off the western coast of Italy in the Mediterranean Sea (a semi-autonomous region of Italy). Several of these cultural patterns were protective against malaria, even when it was endemic to the island, because they minimized exposure or mitigated the consequences of the disease. For example:

- Sardinians were nomadic in a way that reduced exposure to malaria-bearing mosquitos. They grazed flocks of sheep in lowland pastures from November to May, when mosquitos were not active, and returned to higher elevations (where settlements existed and mosquitos less prevalent) in the other, higher risk months.
- Some elements of Sardinian social structure had an impact. Limits on female mobility reduced exposure, because women—especially if pregnant—were largely restricted to the settlement areas, away from the fields. Upper class Sardinians rarely ventured down from higher elevation settlements to the lowland fields, and they selected choice home sites at high locations where the air was cleaner and dryer (and thus had fewer mosquitos). Because they did not typically venture down to the fields, they avoided the warm, moist climate and its higher prevalence of mosquitos.
- The traditional Sardinian ethnomedical system included a belief in hot–cold balance, leading to moderated behavior and the reduction of malaria relapse.

There is also the strange case of avian flu and the cultural attachment to domestic birds. Although avian flu has actually been around for a long time, it first surfaced as a virus that could infect humans in Hong Kong in 1997. The bird flu then spread to Thailand, Vietnam, Indonesia, China, Japan, South Korea, and elsewhere.

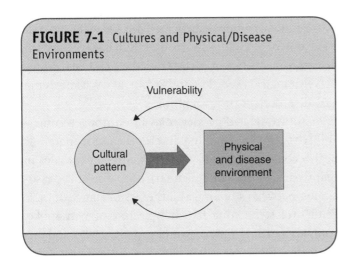

FIGURE 7-1 Cultures and Physical/Disease Environments

In some of these countries, however, poultry is both a major export product (as in, for example, Thailand) and a cultural tradition—most rural homes have chickens, and fighting cocks are prized possessions. In Thailand, a social and cultural conflict ensued when the government tried to implement a mass poultry eradication effort in the countryside to get rid of diseased birds, partly in response to heightened concern by importers of Thai poultry.

Finally, there are potential environmental health consequences of cultural beliefs undergirding profit-driven economic systems, where the natural world is viewed as a resource expressly intended for the use of human beings. This perspective can drive increased risk exposure to pathogens and other health problems, such as:

- Housing and business development that encroaches on forested and natural areas where there are concentrations of parasites or other disease vectors—for example, Lyme disease in the northeastern United States, carried by ticks on wild animals such as deer
- Air and water pollution from unrestricted growth and agricultural or industrial activity, causing increases in respiratory diseases such as asthma and various kinds of cancer, waterborne diseases including cholera, *Escherichia coli* infection, giardiasis, dysentery, or exposure to toxic substances such as arsenic
- Development that destroys natural buffers against severe weather and its human toll—for example, the loss of coastal wetlands and marshland areas that are buffers against floods (such as occurred in August 2005 during Hurricane Katrina in New Orleans), as well as natural ground cover on mountainsides that protects against flooding and mudslides

CULTURAL PATTERNS WITHIN SOCIETIES AND VULNERABILITY TO DISEASE

Now let's look at patterns of vulnerability to disease that are driven by specific internal cultural practices. We have already touched on these in the discussion (Chapter 4) of mental/emotional health and culture-specific syndromes. But culturally specific factors can also create demonstrable vulnerabilities to physical illness. A particular dietary practice, for example, can have potentially serious con-

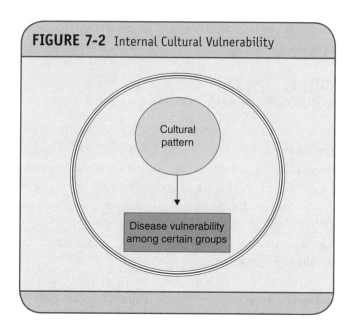

FIGURE 7-2 Internal Cultural Vulnerability

Cultural pattern

Disease vulnerability among certain groups

sequences. One notable example is kuru disease, unique to the Fore tribe in the highlands of Papua New Guinea. Kuru is a fatal and degenerative brain disease (similar to Creutzfeldt-Jakob disease in humans and so-called mad cow disease in cattle). Until the 1950s, a common cultural practice among the Fore was to eat the bodies of the recently deceased as a way of honoring them and returning their spirit to the tribe. There were gender rules involved in this practice: men would eat the meaty, fleshy parts of the body; women and children scooped out and ate the brain tissue. Though the disease was first thought to be hereditary, an American physician discovered that the cause was transmission of malformed proteins called "prions" that eventually caused damage to the host brain. The transmission was directly caused by the funeral cannibalism of the Fore. Once the practice was banned, no children born after the ban developed the disease (information available from the National Institute of Neurological Disorders and Stroke, at www.ninds.nih.gov/disorders/kuru/kuru.htm).

Culture-related gender roles often impact vulnerability to disease. Smoking and tobacco use, and all its health consequences, disproportionally affect males in many parts of the world, primarily because of the association between smoking and the performance of male gender roles. In China, for example, 63% of men smoke, compared to only 3.8% of women (WHO 2003), and this dramatic prevalence gap is typical of several East Asian and Southeast Asian societies. Moreover, in Western societies it is often the case that when women smoke, it is for different reasons than men—for example, as a means of controlling weight (ibid.). The author participated in a study of Southeast Asian immigrants in the United States in which adult Vietnamese viewed the use of cigarettes by women as an indicator of low class and immorality (Edberg et al. 2002).

In northern Kenya, gender-specific iron deficiency is prevalent in some villages, directly attributable to cultural practices. Even in households that are economically self-sufficient, girls are 2.4 times more likely to have iron deficiency as boys. This is due to genderized diet rules in which girls are thought to benefit most from soft foods, such as rice, maize porridge, and tea, while boys are thought to benefit from hard foods such as meat, blood, and beans—the latter far richer in iron (Shell-Duncan and McDade, 2006). Even with further economic development, continuation of this pattern suggests that girls will continue to experience significant iron deficiency (unless there are soft foods that can be added to their diet that are richer in iron).

Anthropologist William Dressler and colleagues (Gravlee, Dressler, & Bernard 2005; Dressler, Balieiro, & Dos Santos 1999; Dressler 1996) have examined cultural beliefs regarding race and their implications for health—on hypertension and blood pressure in particular. In several studies, they have found consistent associations between culturally based race classifications and blood pressure, as opposed to an association between biological skin pigmentation and blood pressure. The method used followed several steps; first to determine culturally specific classifications of race and then to test associations between self-identified racial category (using the classification) and measures of blood pressure. Their research has demonstrated that it is the consequences of discrimination (an issue of cultural values) that do damage, not phenotype (that is, overt, genetically determined skin color).

CULTURE, THE POLITICAL-ECONOMIC ENVIRONMENT, AND DISEASE

The political-economic environment is a broad and complex kind of social ecology. Before we delve into the rela-

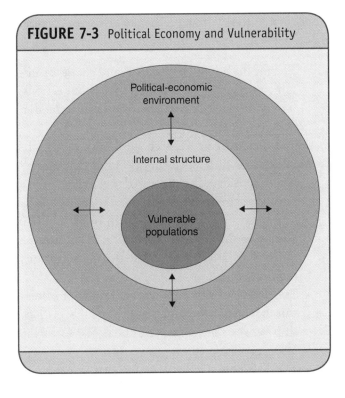

FIGURE 7-3 Political Economy and Vulnerability

tionship between political economy, culture, and health, it should be acknowledged that the general theme of political economy encompasses more than culture, though as explained in Chapter 2, all political and economic systems are infused with cultural ideologies that shape those systems and provide explanation and legitimacy for them. In other words, a free-market economic system is understood to reflect cultural beliefs concerning the free and equal interaction of individuals within a market and the utilitarian goal of the best outcomes for the most people through the mechanism of the market's "invisible hand"[2] that is said to allocate goods and resources in support of this principle. A political system characterized by autocratic monarchy may be understood to reflect a divine hierarchy, such that the monarch is closest to the divine and that his/her commands and use of resources are legitimized above those of any other for that reason.

Most important for our purposes, political economic systems *shape vulnerability* to disease and health problems in general. Why? Because a political economic system includes the way that resources and social benefits are distributed in society, and the nature and logic of

---

[2] From Adam Smith's *The Wealth of Nations* (1776).

the economic activity that produces those resources and goods. This in turn determines:

- The means by which resources and goods are obtained—e.g., through money, social connections, family or clan connections, and entrepreneurial activity.
- The means by which access to health care is obtained and differences in quality of that care. Is health considered a generalized social good, or like any other commodity to be purchased?
- The means by which people can or cannot live a lifestyle that maximizes health. What are the options people have? What do these options require?
- The degree to which people are exposed to stressors that negatively impact health and the relationship between such exposure and access to goods, resources, etc.
- The distribution of social groups that have more or less access to goods, resources, and means to live well, and why the difference in access.
- The types and conditions of work available (or not) in a society and the degree to which different groups of people are exposed to hazards and stressors from these types of work, or to conditions where work is not available.

The logic is inescapable—vulnerability to health problems will generally be higher among those who have the least access and resources. As we discussed Chapter 5, for example, some groups of people are more exposed to the risk of HIV/AIDS than others. Examples include:

- A woman from a poor rural community and a marginalized ethnic group with little access to economic resources comes to an urban setting where sources of income are tough to find, and she exchanges sex for goods or resources because it is necessary—putting her at higher risk for HIV/ AIDS. This is not necessary for individuals who have other means of obtaining resources, but it is for her. She is more vulnerable.
- A man in an urban neighborhood characterized by concentrated poverty, largely cut off from mainstream economic activity, with high levels of vio-

lence and crime is exposed to daily stress levels that are difficult to imagine from the outside. The use of alcohol and drugs as a coping mechanism, and even as a way of maintaining social relationships in that setting, may put the man at very high risk for HIV infection if his drug use includes intravenous drug use.

BOX 7-2 Merrill Singer and Political Economies of Health

Anthropologist Merrill Singer (Center for Health, Intervention and Prevention at the University of Connecticut) has written extensively about health issues of marginalized and high-risk populations in the United States in the context of political economies that structure the context for health. A focus on political economy is central to the perspective known as critical medical anthropology (Baer, Singer, & Susser 2003; Singer & Baer 1995). In brief, critical medical anthropology reframes health issues as embedded in the broader context of inequitable socioeconomic, class, ethnic, and gender relationships. Singer, for example, has linked HIV/AIDS to a litany of other health problems (tuberculosis, infant mortality, hypertension, diabetes, cirrhosis, and substance abuse) that are disproportionately found in poor urban populations, and together calls the aggregate situation "syndemic"—that is, several epidemics that exist together because conditions promote their coexistence (Singer & Clair 2003; Singer 1994). These conditions include poor housing, lack of economic opportunity, racism, violence (at many levels), lack of access to resources, and, generally, lack of access to the tools of power. Continued exposure to such conditions creates a multifaceted vulnerability, in which drug abuse plays a significant role because of its simultaneous qualities of delusion and destruction. As Singer poignantly writes, drug use among the poor is "the medicine that relives but does not heal; the remedy that takes far more than it yields; the lie that embodies all the lies between rich and poor" (2008, 214).

The term *syndemic* was coined by Singer, and there is now a Syndemics Prevention Network at the U.S. Centers for Disease Control and Prevention (www.cdc.gov /syndemics).

Wealth Equity and Inequity as a Key Dimension of Political Economy. It is widely recognized both globally (see WHO 2008) and in the United States that poverty and inequity are major determinants of health. Distributions of wealth, however, are functions of political economy. In the United States, low socioeconomic status (see, for example, Kawachi, Kennedy, & Wilkinson 1999) is widely associated with health risks and problems, such as nutrition, smoking, injuries, environmental pollu-

tion, unemployment, low income, family dysfunction, psychosocial stress, the presence of community violence, limited recreational space, and others. And, the term *Socioeconomic* means more than just income differences. For example, housing segregation by race/ethnicity (regardless of income) is associated with a range of health risks (Williams & Collins 2001; Richards & Lowe 2003, 1171). Neighborhood characteristics (e.g., crime, lack of recreation space) intertwined with socioeconomic status

---

BOX 7-3 Paul Farmer, Philippe Bourgois, Nancy Scheper-Hughes, and the Structural Violence Perspective

Another approach that is essentially political-economic in focus is the idea of structural violence. This refers to systematic aspects of particular social structures—hierarchies, forms of inclusion and exclusion, discrimination, wealth, and resource inequities—that cause harm to some categories of people by denying them access to the benefits of society, including health. Generally, the structural violence perspective (from Galtung 1990; 1969) lays blame on the inequities inherent in the world system; the fact, for example, that there is such a large worldwide gap between rich and poor nations and between rich and poor within nations, and that basic human needs such as health are a commodity—thus subject to whether or not one can afford them. This kind of social injustice is viewed as a form of violence in itself and as a central cause of other forms of violence, including ethnic violence, racial violence, war, and even domestic violence.

Paul Farmer, physician, anthropologist, and founder of the global health and social justice organization, Partners in Health, argues that the factors contributing to human rights violations (violence, torture, rape) are the same factors that create poor health and suffering—inegalitarian societies (Farmer 2003). Victims in these circumstances suffer as a result of structured forces and processes that constrain agency; that is, they limit the ability of individuals to obtain the necessities of life.

Similarly, Nancy Scheper-Hughes and Phillipe Bourgois have both been at the forefront of work illuminating the way that the poor and disenfranchised suffer from daily violence: mothers in Brazil faced with child survival choices, homeless injection drug users, poor people whose organs are used in the illegal organ trade, Salvadorans who experienced brutal military violence during the civil war in the 1980s, young men seeking respect through the only opportunity they see—in the crack cocaine market (Bourgois 1996, 2010; Bourgois, Prince, & Moss 2004; Scheper-Hughes & Bourgois 2004; Scheper-Hughes 1992).

FIGURE 7-4 Man Injecting Drugs

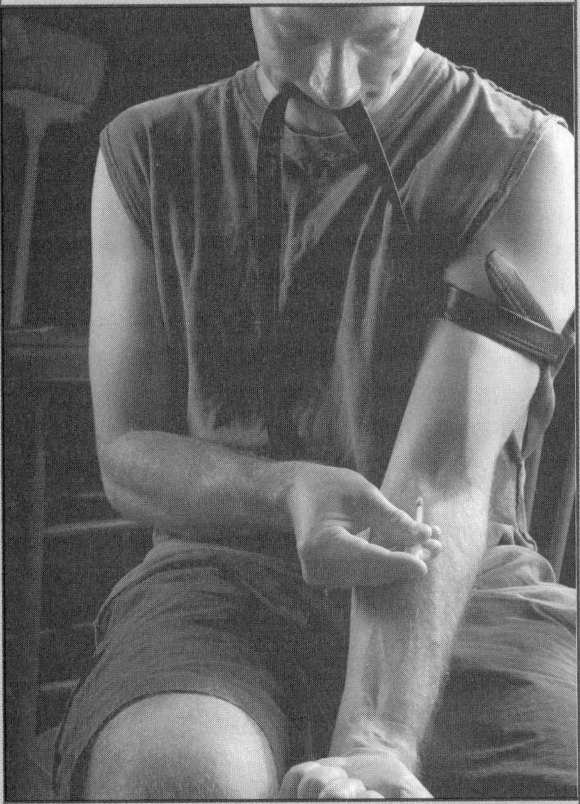

Source: © ejwhite/ShutterStock, Inc.

also have an impact on such health conditions as obesity, violence, and substance use (see Morland et al. 2002; Shihadeh & Flynn 1996; LaVeist & Wallace 2000).

Poverty and social marginalization create groups of people (defined by their socioeconomic status, race/ethnicity, etc.) with poor access to the interrelated systems of health, economic, and social resources. This general access-poor relationship generates patterns of living that focus more on survival and achieving social goals (e.g., family needs, access to resources) within a very limited sphere, as opposed to maximizing health (Sebastian 1999; Sebastian 1996; Flaskerud & Winslow 1998). Such contributing factors to health likely do not operate as distinct factors, but in a co-occurring and interactive fashion, such that a pathway or trajectory with respect to the health of a population is created. Thus socioeconomic status, often linked to historical racism and a legacy of exclusion, shapes a way of life with respect to health that may include not only real limitations on access to and quality of care and higher exposure to community and environmental health risk, but behavior patterns and community norms that follow from expectations of high risk and limited care options and a particular relationship to the healthcare system. What these historical circumstances produce is a trajectory of health for particular populations, which includes their vulnerability and exposure to disease, and the systems of knowledge, attitude, and practice related to health that develops in response to their vulnerability and historical experience within a larger society—or, one could say, a larger environment. This combination of vulnerability, circumstance, and response forms the larger set of forces that, together, create the differences in health status referred to as health disparities.

BOX 7-4 Laura Smith and Political Economy

Think back to the introductory scenario. What might Laura's attitudes towards the healer have to do with political economy? What about her attitudes towards the local patients in the waiting room?

These factors or determinants operate together as a dynamic system over time (Edberg, Cleary, & Vyas 2010; Starfield 2007), shaping an ongoing relationship between a population and the health-related system. The term *health-related system*, in this approach, refers to the combination of health services per se together with the economic, community, social and cultural supports necessary for their effective delivery.

GLOBAL POLITICAL ECONOMIES: GLOBALISM AND COLONIALISM

The political-economic environments to which cultures and societies must respond exist at local, national, regional, and global levels. The overall global economic system is now characterized by globalism. In general, this refers to the way in which the operation of businesses and production is integrated across national boundaries, with global markets and planning across state boundaries. For example, a clothing item is produced in factories in the Philippines in which the workers are both Filipino and migrant Chinese, using cotton that comes from Egypt, and then sold under different brand names at shopping malls in Tokyo, London, and Los Angeles. The whole operation is run by a company headquartered in the United States that is partially owned by a Chinese conglomerate. However, customer service and data processing operations are outsourced to India. As noted in another book in this series (Edberg 2007), globalization in a broader sense refers not just to the integration of economic production and markets, but also to the social and political consequences of this trend. There are many views about whether or not these consequences are positive or negative. For public health, globalization has several implications, including the following:

- Increasing complexity in terms of ensuring workplace health and safety across globalized operations
- Reduced control in any one location concerning labor conditions and the availability of work
- Increasing complexity in terms of ensuring environmental responsibility where facilities and production are segmented and located in different countries, under different regulations and conditions

- Much more rapid routes of transmission for infectious disease around the globe because of the movement of people and goods
- Much more rapid avenues for communication and dissemination
- The increasing juxtaposition of indigenous health systems and biomedical health practices
- As countries develop in broad socioeconomic terms, life expectancy increases and the pattern of morbidity and mortality shifts from infectious disease to lifestyle-related health conditions (e.g., chronic disease, heart disease, cancer). This is known as the *epidemiologic transition* or health transition (see, for example, Omran 1971; Christakis, Ware, & Kleinman 1994)

The economic structure in any one country or region is inevitably tied to the global economic system. This has an impact on health conditions and system capacity. For example, if a country is dependent on just a few export crops subject to the fluctuations of the global market, resources available for health will be uncertain, and long-term planning and services will be less likely. If the economy has shifted to an urban and industrializing economy, with substantial income gaps and decreasing resources outside urban areas, there may be population flows to

FIGURE 7-5 British Explorer Henry Morton Stanley and "Adopted" African Servant Kalulu

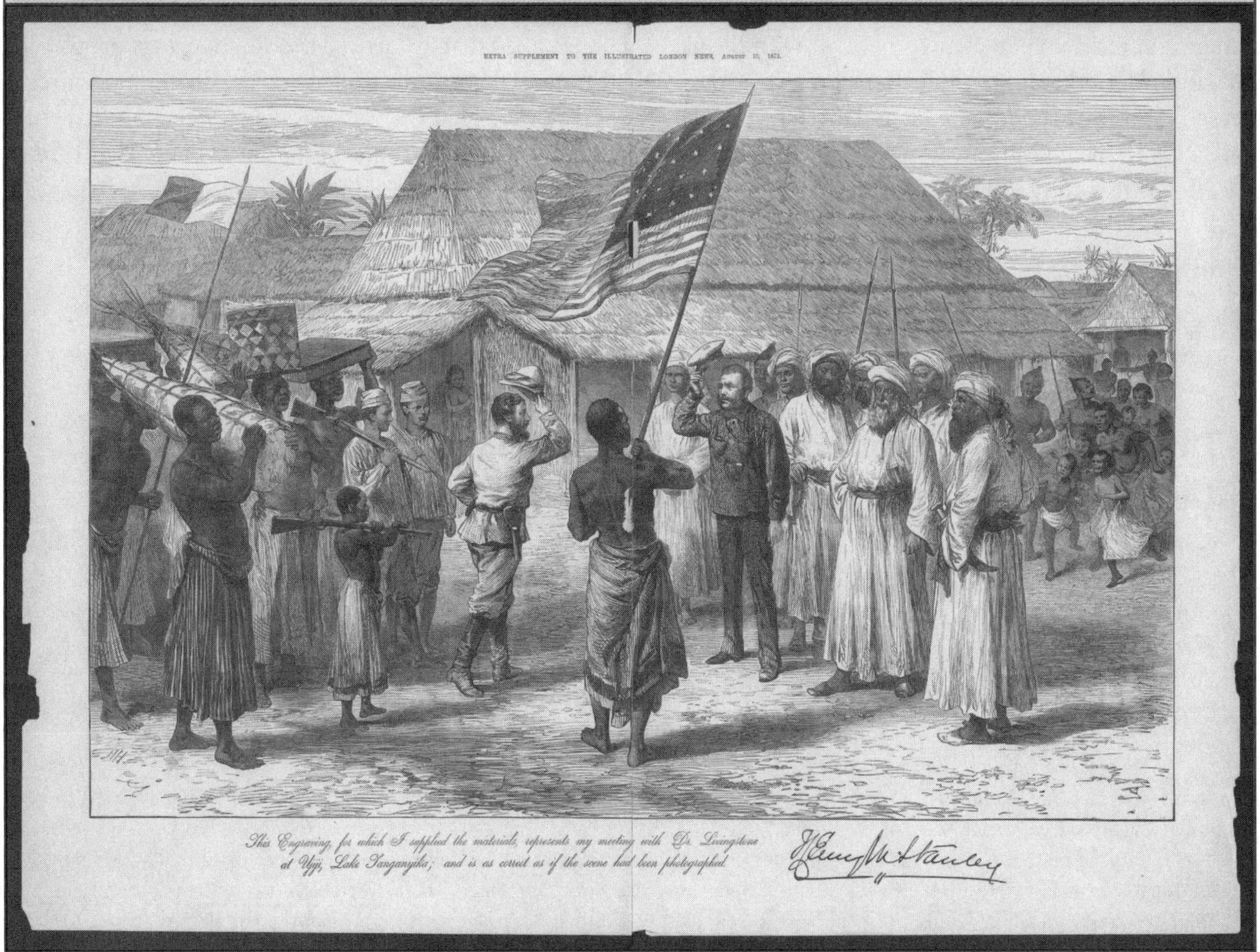

Source: Courtesy of Library of Congress Prints and Photographs Division, [Reproduction number: LC-DIG-ppmsca-18647].

these urban areas leading to crowding, poor living conditions, and the easy transmission of disease. The presence of a highly valued commodity like diamonds, water, or oil may provide the resources to restructure and improve health care; or, it may end up as the source of conflict over resources. In addition, the social structure internal to a country may be significantly affected by globalism, because access to and control over the globalized economic activities in a given country means access to the income generated by those activities. Internal divisions may be exacerbated by this kind of economic polarization, as can be seen in many situations. In the Niger delta region of Nigeria, for example, intense violence in recent years resulted from the immense oil profits gained from Delta oil, while residents of the Delta saw little of that income and suffered from poverty and oil-related pollution.

Globalism is also a major driver of both cultural change and resistance to change, because with the globalization of markets and production comes a vastly increased exposure to goods, media, and lifestyles that may conflict with local cultures, in ways that are perceived as both positive and negative.

Prior to the post–World War II period, these relationships were largely a function of the colonial system, in which production and market relationships were less fluid than they are under the globalized market economy. Under colonialism, the general structure was relatively fixed—Britain, for example, had a defined set of colonies, and the relationship between Britain and these colonies was an economic one (transferring resources to Britain as colonizer) but also a political one, in which the colonies were governed as part of the colonial empire or domain.

In turn, colonies were recognized components of such political domains and also served as bases for extending and maintaining the global power of the colonizer. Within colonies, governing occurred through the intermediary of selected elites overseen by the colonizer (the British model) or by more direct rule carried out by agencies and individuals from the colonizing country (the French model). Either way, a social hierarchy was maintained that influenced the life chances of people, via differential access to education, health care, resources, and power. That hierarchy was typically justified with reference to evolutionary judgments about culture—where the colonizers claimed to represent more advanced cultural forms, bringing civilization to and improving the colonized.

CASE STUDY

Impacts of a Cultural Ecology: Historical Trauma, American Indians/Alaska Natives, and Health

The concept of *historical trauma* has been used in recent years in reference to the health and social effects of long-term population level violence experienced by an entire people as a result of colonialism, slavery, genocide, and other profound historical circumstances. The result of these experiences is often marginalization, poverty, and poor health for these peoples within the context of a broader political-economic system of which they are a part. The social ecology we are talking about, then, involves the relationship between a given population group and the society that structures that historical trauma experience. Cultural patterns related to health for that group evolve out of that relationship, as a process of coping over time (see Starfield 2007; Edberg, Cleary & Vyas 2010).

While historical trauma has also been used regarding Holocaust victims, Japanese survivors of World War II internment camps, and to some extent African Americans, it has most often been used in connection to health issues among American Indian/Alaska native populations in the United States.

The use of historical trauma in this sense has primarily referred to the American Indian experience of chronic, intergenerational trauma and unresolved grief spanning generations, resulting from the genocidal loss of lives, land, and culture from European contact and colonialism (Brave Heart & DeBruyn 1998; Brave Heart-Jordan 1995). As noted earlier (in Chapter 4), historical trauma has poignantly been referred to as a "soul wound" (Duran, Duran, & Yellow Horse Brave Heart 1999). Here is a brief list of key points in that history that relate to the historical trauma experience:

- When the Europeans arrived, there were significant populations of American Indians/Alaska Natives in North America—estimates vary widely, but anywhere from just under 1 million to over 12 million (Lord 1997).
- The native population of the Americas had been there since approximately 12,000 BCE (specific estimates vary on this date), when successive waves of Eurasians came to what is now the United States across the Bering land bridge between Siberia and Alaska called Beringia (now submerged, as the Bering Strait) and expanded throughout North and South America, creating everything from hunter-gatherer societies to the more complex Iroquois and Anasazi (Pueblo) in the United States and the Olmec, Aztec, Maya, and Inca in Central and South America.
- Early on, the relationship between the expanding colonial society in North America and Indian peoples was complex, sometimes involving alliances and collaboration, sometimes involving forced dislocation, conflict, and violence. Indian peoples were, however, typically viewed as uncivilized and subordinate in character to Europeans, and the power of European weaponry enforced an emerging social hierarchy. In addition, native peoples were decimated by diseases such as smallpox brought over from Europe.
- With American independence and rapid population growth, the new country began to expand westward, heightening conflicts over land. In 1830, the Indian Removal Act was passed, authorizing the removal of Indian peoples in the Southeastern states and territories to make way for settlers. This was the setting for the infamous Trail of Tears (Carter 1976), in which some 17,000 Cherokee left or were removed from their homes and 4,000 died during the forced relocation to what is now Oklahoma.
- As settlers moved into the Great Plains and western United States, they met with increased resistance, and there followed a long and violent period of Indian wars between

FIGURE 7-6 World War II Japanese Camp

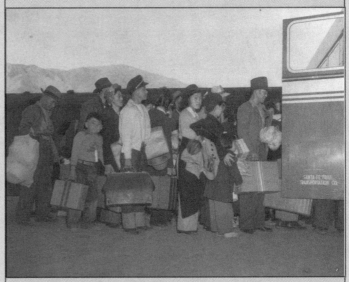

Source: Courtesy of Library of Congress Prints and Photographs Division, [Reproduction number: LC-USZ62-44093].

FIGURE 7-7 Carlisle Indian School (Boarding School)

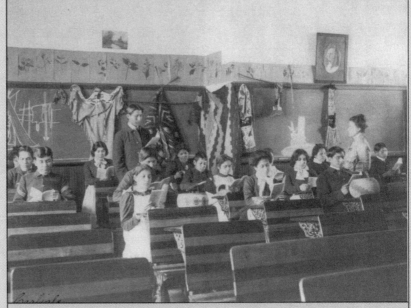

Source: Courtesy of Library of Congress Prints and Photographs Division, Johnston (Francis Benjamin) Collection [Reproduction number: LC-USZ62-47082.]

(Continues)

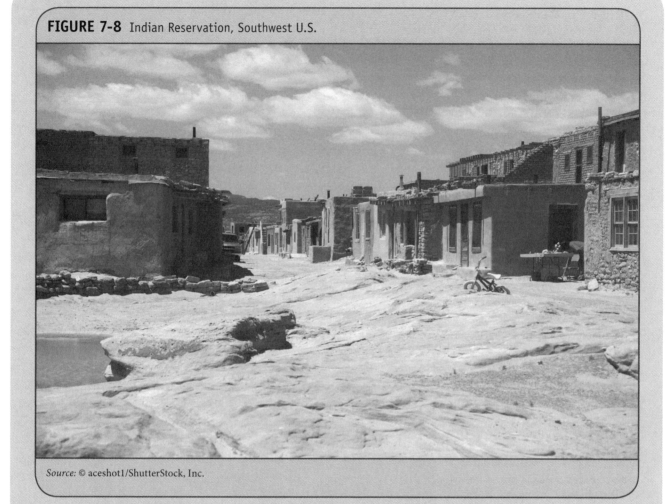

FIGURE 7-8 Indian Reservation, Southwest U.S.

Source: © aceshot1/ShutterStock, Inc.

settlers or the U.S. army and Indian peoples. These conflicts became increasingly brutal, and the army's mission focused on the extermination of Indians who did not surrender and resettle in designated reservations. On these reservations, the land was generally poor, and it was difficult to make a living.

- Following the wars, boarding schools were established with the aim of civilizing and acculturating Indian children by forbidding the practice of their indigenous cultures and religions, prohibiting the use of Indian languages, and often seeking to convert the children to Christianity. Attendance at these boarding schools was common throughout even much of the 20th century, with peak levels in the 1970s. The experience was widely viewed as traumatic.

- Over time, much of the land held by American Indians was appropriated by force or by violating treaties (some was also sold), resulting in the continued loss of both economic and cultural/religious resources. Only in recent years have a number of tribes sued for the return of their lands and been able to control and exploit the resources available to them.

As a result of the long historical experience of colonization, appropriation, cultural suppression, violence, and marginalization, the current situation includes poverty rates twice that of the U.S. population as a whole (U.S. Census Bureau's American Community Survey from 2007 to 2009), and even higher rates

What Is Anomie?

A sociological term popularized (but not originated) by sociologist Emile Durkheim. According to the Random House Dictionary (at www.dictionary.com): "A state or condition of individuals or society characterized by a breakdown or absence of social norms and values, as in the case of uprooted people."

for some tribes such as the Sioux, Navajo, and Apache. Factors related to historical trauma have been associated with a range of social pathologies and negative health/mental health outcomes among American Indians and Alaska Natives (see Struthers and Lowe 2003), such as:

- A high prevalence of cardiovascular disease risk factors such as cigarette smoking and hypertension among American Indians and Alaska Natives, for example, has been related to perceived discrimination and its effects (Krieger, 2000; Johansson, Jacobsen, & Buchwald, 2006).
- Studies have reported strong associations between perceived discrimination and increased depressive symptoms in adult American Indians in the upper Midwest (Whitbeck et al. 2002).
- Loss of self-esteem, depression, poverty, and loss of traditional male roles have been cited as additional factors related to cardiovascular disease (Rhoades 2003).
- Health risk behavior among male American Indians and Alaska Natives may be due to a loss of traditional male roles (Oetting et al. 1998), unresolved grief from historical trauma (Brave Heart & DeBruyn, 1998), and particularly among younger men, anomie and a loss of cultural identity (O'Nell & Mitchell, 1996).

Studies suggest that there is a range of phenomena that may form part of an overall historical trauma syndrome that in turn is associated with numerous health conditions. How does that happen? Whitbeck et al. (2004) made an important contribution by attempting to disentangle the mechanisms through which historical trauma affects American Indians and Alaska Natives. Because the experience was often voiced in terms of *loss*, this important research sought to identify the kinds of losses and resulting emotions associated with historical trauma. Identified losses were converted to items on an historical loss scale and included:

- Loss of land, language, culture, and traditional spiritual ways
- Loss of family ties because of boarding schools; loss of families due to government relocation
- Loss of self-respect due to poor treatment by government officials
- Loss of trust in whites from broken treaties
- Losses from the effects of alcohol
- Loss of respect for elders

FIGURE 7-9 Historical Trauma Model

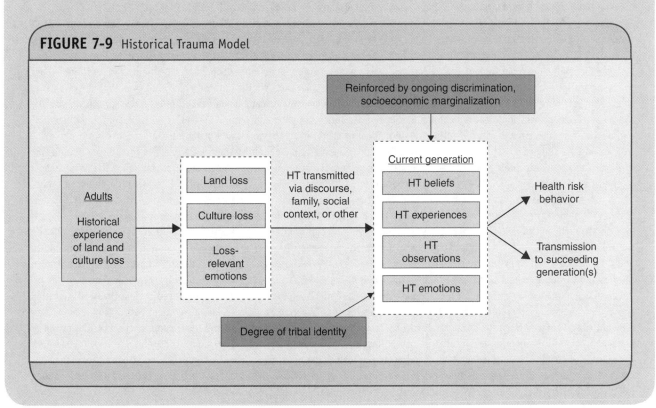

(Continues)

- Loss of people through early death
- Loss of respect by children for traditional ways

   Emotions (symptoms) produced by these losses were then converted to items on an historical loss associated symptoms scale. These included:

- Sadness, depression
- Anger, rage
- Anxiety/nervousness
- Being uncomfortable around white people when thinking of these losses
- Shame when thinking of these losses
- Loss of concentration
- Feeling isolated or distant from other people when thinking of these losses
- Loss of sleep
- Fearful or distrust concerning the intentions of white people
- Feeling like the loss is happening again
- Feeling like avoiding people or places that are reminders of the losses

High loss scores were significantly associated with clusters of emotional symptoms.

   In another significant effort to understand the phenomenon, Evans-Campbell (2008) proposed a multilevel framework for studying the impacts of historical trauma at three levels: individual, family, and community.

1. *Individual* impacts include symptoms characteristic of posttraumatic stress disorder, guilt, anxiety, grief, depression, and other symptoms.

2. At the *family* level, impacts may include impaired family communication and parenting stress.

3. *Community*-level impacts are said to include breakdown of traditional culture and values, loss of traditional rites of passage, alcoholism, physical illness, and internalized racism.

Evans-Campbell also highlighted two key issues regarding historical trauma, as opposed to other kinds of trauma: (1) it is a collective phenomenon, something that happens to a community or a people; and (2) it does not refer to just any kind of trauma, but trauma "perpetrated by outsiders with purposeful and often destructive intent" (ibid., pp. 321).

   These are both significant efforts to identify the specific nature and inherent mechanisms of historical trauma as a political-economic and cultural phenomenon. At the same time, it may be limiting to confine the historical trauma triggers to individual experience with actual land loss, disruption in family systems as a secondary impact, or even loss of specific cultural practices, for example. Many American Indians/Alaska Natives (younger adults, youth) no longer think actively about land loss, the impact of specific historical events, or traditional culture loss. Yet they experience similar/related emotional symptom clusters as do those who attribute their emotions to those issues. It is possible that historical trauma exerts its effect as a broader, socially shared and cross-generational phenomenon, and that to fully understand and address it will require more examination of mediating mechanisms, the ways in which it influences individual interpretation of events, and other indirect impacts.

   All of this suggests that an important dimension of the experience called historical trauma lies in the way people link their own self-image to their perceived social status, in contrast to other segments of society that were once the perpetrators of their historical experience. The self-image aspect refers to identification as a member of an historically oppressed group, and a general, perceived loss of power, control and status. So it isn't just the loss, but the meaning of that loss (what it represents), which in turn has a broad impact on collective, shared psychological experiences of a people.

   In 1969, the anthropologist Anthony Wallace, in his work on cultural destruction and revitalization (much of it focusing on the Iroquois people), described cultural traumas as externally induced stress on the "mazeway"—a mental image people maintain about themselves and their society (Wallace 1969; 1956). Such severe mazeway stressors can result in sociocultural breakdown progressing through various stages, in which cultural well-being and efficacy—the positive, predictive value of culture—is reduced or lost, followed by psychological consequences such as anomie, anxiety, frustration, increased sociopathy. Wallace called these "psychodynamically regressive" responses. While his research occurred some time ago, his general description remains very relevant to the nature of historical trauma. Historical trauma-related cultural beliefs people share about patterns of limitation or negative probability regarding the future, are often played out in day-to-day lived experiences that reinforce the model—e.g., poor health, discrimination, other negative occurrences—as well as the general content of people's conversations and explanations concerning why things are the way they are. So, in response to negative health and social circumstances, Mashpee Wampanoag (a Massachusetts tribe) men say, "Well, that's just part of Mashpee" (Johansson & Doherty 2001).

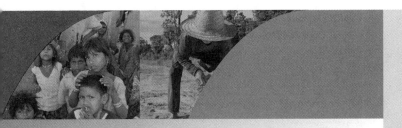

QUESTIONS

1. Can you think of any other internal cultural patterns that cause vulnerabilities to disease?

2. What could the hypothetical Chalmy people do to reduce their malnutrition levels despite the constraints they face?

3. What are some political-economic circumstances that could impede people from engaging in exercise as prevention for diabetes and cardiovascular disease?

4. What could be done to reduce the health consequences of historical trauma?

REFERENCES

Baer, H.A., M. Singer, and I. Susser. 2003. *Medical Anthropology and the World System*, 2nd ed. Westport, CT: Praeger Publishers.

Bourgois, P. 1996. *In Search of Respect: Selling Crack in El Barrio.* Cambridge, MA: Cambridge University Press.

Bourgois, P. 2010. "Recognizing Invisible Violence: A 30-year Ethnographic Retrospective." In *Global Health in Times of Violence*, edited by B. Rylko-Bauer, P. Farmer, and L. Whiteford, 17–40. Santa Fe, NM: School for Advanced Research Press.

Bourgois, P., B. Prince, and A. Moss. 2004. "Everyday Violence and the Gender of Hepatitis C among Homeless Drug-Injecting Youth in San Francisco." *Human Organization* 63 (3): 253–264.

Brave Heart, M.Y.H., and L.M. DeBruyn. 1998. "The American Indian Holocaust: Healing Historical Unresolved Grief." *American Indian and Alaska Native Mental Health Research* 8 (2): 56–78.

Brave Heart-Jordan, M.Y.H. 1995. *The Return to the Sacred Path: Healing from Historical Trauma and Historical Unresolved Grief among the Lakota.* Unpublished doctoral dissertation. Smith College, Northampton, MA.

Brown, P. 2010/1998. "Cultural Adaptations to Endemic Malaria in Sardinia." In *Understanding and Applying Medical Anthropology*, 2nd ed., edited by P. Brown and R. Barrett, pp. 79–92. New York: McGraw-Hill.

Carter, S. 1976. *Cherokee Sunset: A Nation Betrayed: A Narrative of Travail and Triumph, Persecution and Exile.* New York: Doubleday.

Christakis NA, Ware NC, and Kleinman AM. 1994. "Illness Behavior and the Health Transition in the Developing World." In L.C. Chen, A.M. Kleinman, J. Potter, J. Caldwell, and N.C. Ware (Eds), *Health and Social Change in International Perspective.* Boston, MA: Harvard University Press.

Diamond, J. 1999. *Guns, Germs, and Steel: The Fates of Human Societies.* New York: W.W. Norton & Co.

Dressler, W.W. 1996. "Culture and Blood Pressure: Using Consensus Analysis to Create a Measurement." *Field Methods* 1996: 6–8.

Dressler, W.W., M.C. Balieiro, and J.E. Dos Santos. 1999. "Culture, Skin Color and Arterial Blood Pressure in Brazil." *American Journal of Human Biology* 11 (1): 49–59.

Duran, B., E. Duran, and M. Y. H. Brave Heart. 1999. "Native Americans and the Trauma of History." In *Studying Native America: Problems and Prospects*, edited by R. Thornton, pp. 60–76. Social Science Research Council, American Indian Studies Advisory Panel. Madison, WI: University of Wisconsin Press.

Edberg, M., S. Cleary, and A. Vyas. February 2010. "A Model for Understanding and Assessing Health Disparities in Immigrant/Refugee Communities." *Journal of Immigrant and Minority Health.* DOI 10.1007/s10903-010-9337-5.

Edberg, M. 2007. *Essentials of Health Behavior: Social and Behavioral Theory in Public Health.* Boston: Jones and Bartlett Publishers.

Edberg, M., F. Wong, R. Park, and K. Corey. 2002, July. "Preliminary Qualitative Results from an Ongoing Study of HIV Risk in Three Southeast Asian Communities." *Proceedings of the XIV International AIDS Conference*, Barcelona, Spain: World Health Organization, UNAIDS, Centers for Disease Control and other sponsors.

Evans-Campbell, T. 2008. "Historical Trauma among American Indian/Native Alaska Communities: A Multilevel Framework for Exploring Impacts on Individuals, Families and Communities." *Journal of Interpersonal Violence* 23: 316–338.

Farmer, P. 2003. *Pathologies of Power: Health, Human Rights, and the New War on the Poor.* Berkeley, CA: University of California Press.

Flaskerud, J.H., and B.J. Winslow. 1998. "Conceptualizing Vulnerable Populations Health-Related Research." *Nursing Research* 47 (2): 69–78.

Galtung, J. 1969. "Violence, Peace and Peace Research." *Journal of Peace Research* 6 (3): 167–191.

Galtung, J. 1990. "Cultural Violence." *Journal of Peace Research* 27 (3): 291–305.

Gravlee, C.C., W.D. Dressler, and H.R. Bernard. 2005. "Skin Color, Social Classification and Blood Pressure in Southeastern Puerto Rico." *American Journal of Public Health* 95: 2191–2197.

Johansson, P., and O. Doherty. 2001, March/April. *Mashpee Wampanoag Tribe Talking Circles.* Unpublished report.

Johansson, P., C. Jacobsen, and D. Buchwald. 2006. "Perceived Discrimination in Healthcare among American Indians/Alaska Natives." *Ethnicity and Disease* 16 (4), 766–771.

Kawachi, I., B.P. Kennedy, and R.G. Wilkinson. 1999. *Society and Population Health Reader, Volume I: Income Inequality and Health.* New York: The New Press.

Krieger, N. 2000. "Discrimination and Health." In *Social Epidemiology*, edited by L. Berkman and I. Kawachi, 36–75. Oxford, England: Oxford University Press.

LaVeist, T.A., and J.M. Wallace. 2000. "Health Risk and the Inequitable Distribution of Liquor Stores in African-American Neighborhoods." *Social Science and Medicine* 51: 613–17.

Lord, L. 1997. "How Many People Were Here before Columbus?" *US News and World Report* August 18–25, pp. 68–70.

Morland, K., S. Wing, A. Diez-Roux, and C. Poole. 2002. "Neighborhood Characteristics Associated with Location of Food Stores and Food Service Places." *American Journal of Preventive Medicine* 22: 23–29.

Oetting, E.R., J.F. Donnermeyer, J.E. Trimble, and F. Beauvais. 1998. "Primary Socialization Theory: Culture, Ethnicity, and Cultural Identification. The Links between Culture and Substance Use IV." *Substance Use & Misuse* 33 (10): 2075–2107.

Omran AR. 1971. "The Epidemiological Transition: A Theory of the Epidemiology of Population Change." *Milbank Memorial Fund Quarterly* 49: 509–538.

O'Nell, T.D., and C.M. Mitchell. 1996. "Alcohol Use among American Indian Adolescents: The Role of Culture in Pathological Drinking." *Social Science & Medicine* 42 (4): 565–578.

Rhoades, E.R. 2003. "The Health Status of American Indian and Alaska Native Males." *American Journal of Public Health* 93 (5): 774–778.

Richards, C.F., and R.A. Lowe. 2003. "Researching Racial and Ethnic Disparities in Health." *Academy of Emergency Medicine* 10 (11): 1169–1175.

Scheper-Hughes, N. 1992. *Death without Weeping: The Violence of Everyday Life in Brazil.* Berkeley: University of California Press.

Scheper-Hughes, N., and P. Bourgois, Eds. (2004). *Violence in War and Peace: An Anthology.* Oxford, England: Blackwell Publishing.

Sebastian, J.G. 1996. "Vulnerability and Vulnerable Populations." In *Community Health Nursing: Promoting the Health of Individuals, Aggregates and Communities,* 4th ed., edited by M. Stanhope and J. Lancaster. St. Louis, MO.: Mosby.

Sebastian, J.G. 1999. "Definitions and Theory Underlying Vulnerability." In *Special Populations in the Community: Advances in Reducing Health Disparities,* edited by J.G. Sebastian and A. Bushy. Gaithersburg, MD: Aspen Publications.

Shell-Duncan, B., and T. McDade. 2006. "The Cultural Ecology of Iron Deficiency among Northern Kenyan Schoolchildren." *Journal of Human Ecology* Special Issue 14: 107–116.

Shihadeh, E.S., and N. Flynn. 1996. "Segregation and Crime: The Effect of Black Isolation on the Rates of Black Urban Violence." *Sociological Forces* 74: 1325–1352.

Singer, M. 1994. "AIDS and the Health Crisis of the U.S. Urban Poor: The Perspective of Critical Medical Anthropology." *Social Science and Medicine* 39 (7): 931–948.

Singer, M. 2008. *Drugging the Poor: Legal and Illegal Drugs and Social Inequality.* Long Grove, IL: Waveland Press, Inc.

Singer, M., and H.A. Baer. 1995. *Critical Medical Anthropology.* Amityville, NY: Baywood Publishing.

Singer, M., and S. Clair. 2003. "Syndemics and Public Health: Reconceptualizing Disease in Bio-Social Context." *Medical Anthropology Quarterly* 17 (4): 423–441.

Starfield, B. 2007. "Pathways of Influence on Equity in Health." *Social Science and Medicine* 64: 1355–1362.

Struthers, R. and J. Lowe. 2003. "Nursing in the Native American Culture and Trauma." *Issues in Mental Health Nursing* 24: 257–272.

U.S. Census Bureau. *2007–2009 American Community Survey 3-Year Estimates.* Washington, DC: U.S. Census Bureau.

Wallace, A.F.C. 1956. "Revitalization Movements." *American Anthropologist* 58: 264–281.

Wallace, A.F.C. 1969. *The Death and Rebirth of the Seneca.* New York: Vintage Books.

Whitbeck, L.B., G.W. Adams, D.R. Hoyt, and X. Chen. 2004. "Conceptualizing and Measuring Historical Trauma among American Indian People." *American Journal of Community Psychology* 33 (3/4): 119–130.

Whitbeck, L.B., B.J. McMorris, D.R. Hoyt, J.D. Stubben, and T. Lafromboise. 2002. "Perceived Discrimination, Traditional Practices, and Depressive Symptoms among American Indians in the Upper Midwest." *Journal of Health & Social Behavior* 43 (4): 400–418.

WHO. 2003, November. *Gender, Health and Tobacco.* From Gender and Health Information Sheet series. Geneva, Switzerland: World Health Organization. Accessed at www.who.int/gender /documents/Gender_Tobacco_2.pdf

WHO. 2008. *Closing the Gap in a Generation: Health Equity through Action on the Social Determinants of Health. Final Report of the Commission on Social Determinants of Health.* Geneva, Switzerland: World Health Organization.

Williams, D.R., and C. Collins. 2001. "Racial Residential Segregation: A Fundamental Cause of Racial Disparities in Health." *Public Health Reports* 116 (5): 404–416.

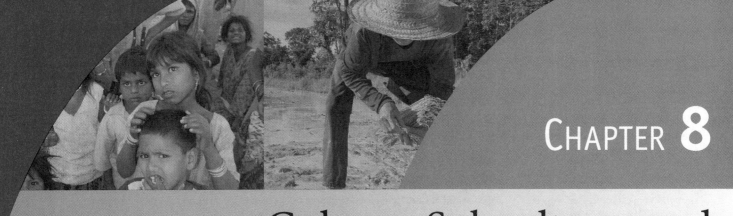

CHAPTER 8

Culture, Subculture, and Constructions of Health Risk

"People select their awareness of certain dangers to conform with a specific way of life . . . To alter risk selection and risk perception, then, would depend on changing the social organization."

—Mary Douglas and Aaron Wildavsky (1982, 9).

"Each form of social life has its own typical risk portfolio. Common values lead to common fears . . . Risk taking and risk aversion, shared confidence and shared fears, are part of the dialogue on how best to organize social relations."

—Ibid., 8

Here are some simple truisms, of a sort. Working from a public health perspective, certain kinds of behaviors, social practices, or beliefs are easily called "risky" or "at risk" if they present risks for infection, injury, physical functioning, or other biomedical health conditions. True enough.

The dilemma for this chapter is that human beings don't always—and possibly just sometimes—factor actual health risk into calculations about what to do or not do. One reason should be clear from all that has been covered so far in this book: there are different definitions of health, and these definitions may or may not align with a strict biomedical construction. The second reason should also be clear by now: Health, however defined, is

still just one kind of motivation or determining factor underlying behavior. Gender, status, economic need, moral codes, and all kinds of other factors may trump health concerns, or even concerns about physical safety and injury (Douglas & Wildavsky 1982; Douglas 1992; Tansey & O'Riordan 1999). So, if you are working as a practitioner or researcher with a general goal of maximizing health, you are more likely to help in achieving a useful outcome if you enter a given situation with these truisms in mind. There is a great diversity of human circumstances out there, and assuming that one logic fits all is not going to be productive most of the time.

That said, let's take a look at some case examples of how considerations of health risk (and in these examples, significant risk) are shaped by multiple factors.

RITES OF PASSAGE AND HEALTH RISK

All cultures include *rites of passage* as part of the process of moving from one stage in life to another, whether initiation into adulthood, marriage, funerals, or other stages (see Van Gennep 1909; Turner 1969). These rites involve ceremonies, but also in some cases trials that the initiate must undergo to demonstrate readiness to move to the next phase. This is true, for example, with many rites of passage to manhood and womanhood. Van Gennep (ibid.) wrote that such rituals involve a separation from society, a liminal (in-between) phase, where initiates may undergo symbolic death, be separated or

TABLE 8-1 Social/Cultural Factors Affecting Perceived Risk—Examples

(Public health perspective) risk behavior	Mediating social/cultural factors	Primary perceived risk (by specific individuals)
Low condom use (among sex workers)—risk of HIV/sexually transmitted infection	Social and cultural obligation to support family	Risk of not earning income to provide for family
Preparing/serving foods high in fat—risk for obesity, diabetes, poor cardiovascular health	Culturally important foods to maintain social role and identity	Risk of losing social standing, losing identity
Youth involved in violence—risk of injury or fatality	Role of violence in symbolizing power and esteemed social role	Risk of victimization, low social status, low access to resources

CASE 8-1

Runaway Youth and HIV/AIDS

By now everyone ought to know that HIV/AIDS is a serious, potentially fatal, though now at least manageable, condition (and the manageable part only became true after the mid to late 1990s). It would seem logical to try to avoid actions that put oneself at high risk for HIV transmission—but of course, we know that is not the operating logic much of the time, or HIV/AIDS would not be as prevalent as it is. In the 1990s, I worked on a study funded by the National Institute on Drug Abuse to assess the substance abuse and HIV/AIDS risk patterns of runaway youth, considered to be a general population at high risk for AIDS (Edberg 1994). The study was conducted in multiple cities in order to capture a range of runaway youth subcultures and circumstances. In the Washington, DC, and Baltimore, Maryland, areas, I accessed three subgroups of homeless and runaway youth—which was only a subset of the different categories of youth in that situation. The three groups included: African American youth primarily from the southeast quadrant of Washington, DC; runaway youth in the Baltimore area who were primarily from working class and immigrant families; and punk/skinhead runaways in certain areas of the northwest quadrant in Washington, DC, primarily from middle/upper class families and who had run from a considerable distance (other states).

The research effort involved an extensive structured interview on drug use and substance use, as well as open-ended, qualitative questions concerning home situations, social support, how the youth survived out of their homes, and other questions about living patterns. The research was also ethnographic, involving a considerable amount of time in various settings where runaways were (in shelters, on the streets, in stores and commercial areas, and in clubs).

The Punks/Skinheads

This was the early 1990s, and in Washington, DC, the tail end of a punk/skinhead youth culture was still evident, though not nearly as prominent as it had been in the early and mid-1980s, when the ("harDCcore") scene gave birth to such seminal bands as Black Flag (Henry Rollins), Minor Threat, Bad Brains, and later Fugazi, as well as the local record company Dischord Records, and punk political activism was exemplified by the Positive Force group (see Andersen and Jenkins 2003). But youth who ran away from home or were forced out of the Washington, DC, suburbs or from other states still continued to go to Washington, DC, because they heard that there might be friendly faces and people who would understand them. These were runaways in the classic sense, youth who thought of themselves as misfits, though most came from at least middle class homes if not homes that were wealthier. This was not the case for some of the other runaway groups I interviewed.

Youth in this category were primarily Caucasian, and they were not just on the street in transition between staying with extended family or fictive kin[1] type relations (as with many of the African American runaways). They came from afar because

---

[1] *Fictive kin* refers to a relationship between people who are not technically family, but who are treated (and sometimes talked about) as if they are.

of the expectation of an underground peer network, and for the most part that is what they found. At the same time, their situations were precarious, because they sometimes lived in abandoned houses or buildings called "squats," or stayed temporarily with someone, or lived under bridges and other such locations. They panhandled for food or engaged in petty theft. Some engaged in survival sex, selling themselves as needed. Some sold small quantities of drugs within the social network. Of all the three categories of runaways, this group had the highest drug use prevalence—reporting use of marijuana, LSD, over-the-counter drugs, methamphetamine, heroin, inhalants, crack, and others, as well as large amounts of alcohol. They also came from households where there was some level of family dysfunction if not actual abuse—a few reported what appeared to be substantial physical abuse.

Several of the respondents in this category pointedly differentiated themselves from popular characterizations of skinheads, rejecting racism and calling themselves "unity skinheads." In keeping with the political activism of the punk movement in the district at the time, they also appeared to share a general set of anarchist beliefs, though not well defined, along with beliefs about conspiracies regarding the way the world was governed and concerns about the police state, racism, nuclear war, and other related issues. One of the respondents in this category, Buzz (a pseudonym, as with all the names in this case study), said "There are a lot of runaways who are against the system, so you can either use it for your own ends or stay out of it. I got food stamps once, but only for a couple of weeks, and only because the people where I was staying asked me to help them . . . No, I take care of myself."

Another youth, Carol, said, "I believe that society first blames the blacks for everything that's going around, and then they come to like the punks and freaks like us. And then blame it on us, when there's no one else to blame it on, which is usually wrong."

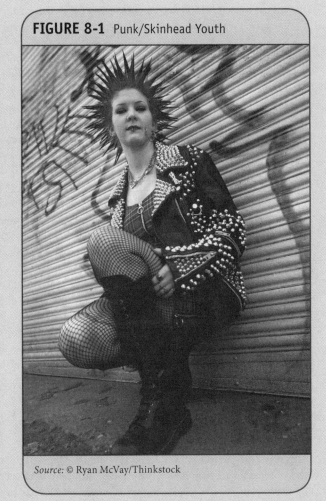

FIGURE 8-1 Punk/Skinhead Youth

Source: © Ryan McVay/Thinkstock

Though different in socioeconomic background from the other categories of runaways interviewed, the punk/skinheads still faced a dangerous existence on the streets and at times felt that their life span was limited. To compensate, these runaways relied heavily on peer networks for survival, which also had an impact on who they thought of as potentially risky sex partners for transmission of HIV or other sexually transmitted infections. The text segment that follows is from an interview with an 18-year-old punk runaway on the street, illustrating the strong connection with peers in that subculture:

Mainly my homeless experience was with skinheads and punk rockers, and there's a camaraderie between them. If they cannot eat half their dinner and [can] sneak it out to you, they will. If they've got 10 bucks and you're hungry, they'll take you out to like Tasty Diner, it's only $2.50 for some ham and eggs. But it's food and you've got it. And if there's beer, they'll share it, and if the cops come, and you get busted for something they did, or whatever, they'll take up for you. I've seen that happen, and it's more than just a friendly camaraderie, it's like family. And I think that the government doesn't understand skinheads. They think that they're all Nazis. But if it wasn't for skinheads, I'd probably be dead or a prostitute, or both. A dead prostitute. They took me in. They were my friends. They helped me find jobs. They cut my hair weird, but they were good people. They didn't leave me for dead in the streets. They weren't like, "Well, my parents won't like it." They were like, "f___ my parents, we'll sneak in the basement window. You can't sleep out on the street.

(Continues)

It's snowing. It's raining," you know, or, "It's cold out tonight. Here you can have my favorite sweater. It will keep you warm. You want some clean socks, here's some clean socks. You want to do your laundry here, it's free."

The actual reported risk behavior for HIV/AIDS was related to both drug and alcohol use and to sex. While only two of the runaways in this category had injected drugs, there was some indication of the assumption of safety among the group even among these respondents. A 17-year-old respondent we will call "Sue" was asked whether she cleaned her needles or used fresh ones and she replied: "No, I don't bother . . . I don't see any reason for it. There's no point 'cause I trust the people I share it with. It's just a waste of time." These runaways tended to have high numbers of sex partners because it was common to meet someone in a club, sleep with them for a place to stay, and then move on and repeat the pattern. Two respondents had sex for money on occasion. With a few exceptions, condom use was low, even though knowledge of HIV risk was high. Reasons for the risk varied from not caring to feeling safe because sex partners were primarily people they knew. Alyssa (age 18) said that she worried about AIDS, but that she was "a little cleaner than most people" and steered clear of people who were "junkies, sluts, or a real dirtbag about sleeping with people." She also got tested for HIV. Alice (age 15) never used condoms, but didn't feel like she was at risk for HIV/AIDS because "the people that I would do something with I know or know things about . . ."

Construction of Risk for HIV/AIDS. The rationale expressed about risk for HIV/AIDS reflected their situation. Out on the street, confronted by hunger, lack of shelter, and extreme vulnerability to exploitation or other risks, what priority would be placed on risk for HIV/AIDS? It had to be weighed against other concerns and motivations. Some of these motivating factors were not related to competing risks and dangers, but to the generalized political worldview that was part of the punk/skinhead subculture, reinforced by compelling peer bonds. So, even if one of these youth had the *intent* to get an HIV test, or to get treatment for a sexually transmitted infection, he or she had no insurance or medical provider and resisted going to any health provider or clinic that did not understand his or her political rejection of the dominant hierarchy of wealth and profit. For the most part, it meant that free clinics were the only alternative—and there were only a few of those. More important, it became clear in the interviews that there was an "in group-out group" differentiation made in terms of who was considered to be a risky sexual partner. In short, most people within the subculture were generally seen as clean, while outsiders were not.

So the judgment of risk was based on *subcultural affinity*—and no wonder. Connections with the peer group were so important for survival that maintaining a solid relationship governed many decisions. Who would want to alienate someone in the group by suspecting him of being risky or unclean as a sex partner? The general sentiment was "The world is against us," and so "my friends are all there is" (much like the ethic of soldiers in battle). Therefore, few risks outweighed preservation of that social unit. Given that worldview, it might have been useful to channel HIV prevention efforts through one or more of the local, informal punk houses that had evolved into centers of activity (at the time of this research), organizing outdoor music and fundraisers for free clinics and other causes. These houses (e.g., Positive Force) could potentially mobilize networks of friends who shared a misfit or rebel identity, and messages could include themes about protecting friends (see also Edberg 2007, Chapter 12).

in seclusion, or may have to undergo a particularly risky experience. When a risky situation is part of the ritual process, it will be interpreted with a very different lens than just thinking about the risk alone. Where a public health approach aims to prevent or avoid risk, some rites of passage assume that pain or potential danger are necessary elements of the transition. Consider these examples:

- *The complicated issue of female circumcision (genital cutting):* According to the World Health Organization, approximately 92 million girls from age 10 and older have undergone this ritual.[1] It is viewed in a number of cultures—including those in central and northeast Africa, in some Middle Eastern societies, and Indonesia in Southeast Asia—as necessary for a girl to be ready for marriage, and for her to be seen as properly feminine, modest, and clean, and as a means of controlling sexual behavior. Yet its health consequences can be serious, including urinary infections, infertility,

---

[1] WHO refers to the practice as "Female Genital Mutilation" and considers it a violation of human rights.

CASE 8-2

Girls at Risk for Sex Trade Involvement

The author was also involved in a study assessing the circumstances of girls and young women at risk for or involved in the sex trade—clearly a high-risk situation for HIV/AIDS, sexually transmitted infections, and violence. Surveys were conducted with girls who participated in a San Francisco, California–based intervention program, and extended qualitative interviews were conducted with a smaller subgroup of these participants. Interviews were also conducted with program staff (Cohen, Edberg, & Gies 2010). From the interviews, four pathways of involvement in commercial sex emerged, forming a rough typology:

- *Type 1. Girls/Young Women from Risk-Saturated Communities:* Concentrated poverty, urban communities, with multiple risks.
- *Type 2. Girls/Young Women from Troubled Suburban Families:* Family dysfunction and dislocation were more typically the contributing factors, as opposed to community.
- *Type 3. Girls/Young Women from Immigrant Families:* Risks related to generational conflict, language and culture barriers.
- *Type 4. Girls/Young Women Proactively Involved:* Primarily related to higher end commercial sex, less emphasis on survival need.

These typologies are of course not exact—some girls/young women shared characteristics of more than one typology. But they are useful abstractions and help in understanding how involvement and the associated risks are understood. For this discussion, we will focus on girls in the type 1 category, characterized more specifically as:

- From high-poverty, high-risk communities. Multiple, syndemic risks such as violence, drugs, dealing, family disruption, domestic violence, pimps as part of community. No one risk is definitive.
- Commercial sex is not an outlier in such circumstances but an extension of many exploitative relationships. In such communities, commercial sex appears to be part of a continuum of activities that are inherent to the socioeconomic pattern, the street economy.
- Risk behaviors, including sex for goods/money, are normalized.
- Girls/young women in this trajectory become involved with intervention programs at relatively young age, by multiple paths, not necessarily due to commercial sex involvement.

In this category, sex risk is most clearly framed against shared understandings among many individuals in risk-saturated communities about relationship between those risks and all the others that are present, creating a stark assessment of relative risk. Girls from risk-saturated communities appeared to view sex for money as part of a much broader pattern of exchanging whatever one had available for money or resources. It was something they had often seen since they were little, and it was reinforced by a prevalent pimp culture in which pimps, and the lifestyle, were glamorized. Because these communities were saturated with so many risks, a kind of community culture developed in which expectations were limited about the likelihood of positive options. Because of that, many situations that would otherwise be seen as unacceptable were normalized.

In the interview segment that follows, a young girl in this category talks about her recruitment into commercial sex. As you read this interview excerpt, remember that she was just 14 when these events took place. It is remarkable for the ordinary discourse through which an otherwise extraordinary series of actions and circumstances are treated:

> I was skipping school, just being bad, doing what I wanted to do, smoking weed, just popping pills, and then 1 day I was walking down by Lowell in Mission [in San Francisco], walking down towards Geneva, and I was gonna go pay my phone [bill], and a big ol' car rolled up. It was a Camaro, a candy-cane [red] Camaro with like 22-inch rims. . . . And he was like: "What's up? How you doing? Where are you going?" And he double parked the car, got out the car, and wanted to talk to me, so I started talking to him cuz he wasn't ugly. Like he was tall, light skin, black guy, green eyes, he opened his mouth and a bunch of diamonds in his mouth, big ol' chain, I was like . . . wow. So he came up to me, he was like, "My name is [deleted]." I was like, "What's up, my name is [deleted]." And then he was like, "Oh, why don't you give me your number," and whatever. And I was like, "All right." So I gave it to him, and then he called and whatever, after I paid my phone bill. . . . He called me and whatever, and he was like, "Oh, we're having a get together with my friends," and I didn't know he was talking about his friends as in his ho's [whores]. So he was like, "We are having a get together at this

hotel right by your house, the Mission Inn, right down on Lowell." And I was like, "Oh, OK," and I showed and whatever and he was just like, "I don't know." He was all trying to get at me like a boyfriend–girlfriend type a way, and then I was just taken, like stupid, cuz he was just so cute.

The pimp she was referring to was 25 years old. And at that point, she was not attending school. "I wanted more money at that time," she said. "So, I was already at the point of what should I do, start selling dope? Or what should I do?" She was getting money from her mother, but "I didn't want to ask her no more."

At the Mission Inn, the same night:

> And then after, he [the pimp] was like, "Do you like making money?" And I was like, "Yeah, I like money, who doesn't?" Right? Then he was like, "You should get in this business with me." I was like, "What kind of business?" And he was like," You know what kind of business." I was like, "No, really, I don't know what kind of business." And he was like, "Well, it's like escorting business." I was like, "Oh, OK." I was like still clueless. "What is that?" He was like, "Well, I'm gonna have my friend tell you about it and then you will see if you like it. If you don't, then you don't have to do it." And then I was like, "All right," and then we had a call that same night, and she was like, "Oh, I have my friend with me to the trick." She was like, "Oh, I have a friend with me, you should try both of us," or whatever. And then we went. . . .

By 2:00 a.m., she was put out on the street—the "track"—to solicit.

Another girl in this category talked about a time when she was attacked while involved in commercial sex in Las Vegas. She was 12 years old at the time. The attack took her by surprise—because she was accustomed to all the characters in her world "knowing the rules." She explained it as follows:

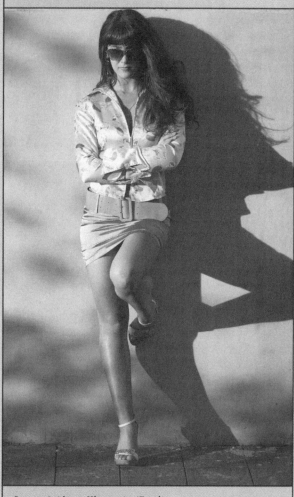

FIGURE 8-2 Girl at Risk for Sex Trade Involvement

Source: © Alexey Klementiev/Fotolia

> [W]hen I was doing it, it really didn't come to mind that something would happen to me like that. You know, cuz it was like, a ho know what role a ho is suppose to play. A pimp know what role a pimp is suppose to play. A trick know what role a trick is suppose to play. You know, we all know what role we are suppose to play. We all know how to work our business, you know, from a money-making point of view. Ask me from a pimp's point of view how he should run his, and even from a trick, how a trick know how he's suppose to get pleased. Things like that. You know, sometimes you do get those tricks out there that don't want to pay you. That don't want to play his role that he's suppose to play. Like I said when I was doing it, it was like, OK, it was smooth. I didn't have no problem. You know, the guys knew what they were suppose to do and blah, blah, blah.

The Role of Pimps in Risk-Saturated Communities. The role of pimps is a constant factor in many of the interviews with girls in the risk-saturated category. Pimps are talked about as a feature of the communities from which the girls/young women are involved. To summarize simply what these preliminary data suggest: In saturated high-risk communities, the pimp's social role intersects with the culture of glamour and money that is associated with prostitution. Moreover, in these communities, pimps not only play to that role, but sometimes set up a form of "household," composed of a number of women, who may be age graded, where an older prostitute in the household sometimes helps in recruiting, clothing, and training younger girls. The relationship between any of these girls/women and the pimp is complicated, sometimes verging on a boyfriend-type relationship, sometimes abusive, and yet centered on the money brought in, the minimum expected role for the girls. There is competition between pimps, and girls are sometimes recruited out of another pimp's group, for which there may be reprisals. At the same time, pimps seem to make most of the arrangements in terms of posting on the Internet, driving girls around, recruiting, and handling all the money. Most of the young respondents seemed accustomed to giving the pimp all or most of their earnings. Several of the respondents in this category were also clearly attracted to the glamour and money associated with the image.

What Is the Risk? Again, the question is, given the subculture created within these communities of concentrated poverty and marginalization, what would be viewed as a risk in this situation? Potential violence? Transmission of HIV or a sexually transmitted infection? Dropping out of school? Maybe all of them would be acknowledged as risks in some way, but compared to basic needs for resources, even the perception of an ongoing connection to a social unit where money is involved may outweigh those concerns. The others may be seen as risks, but as relative risks.

childbirth complications, and mortality (WHO 2010).

- *Drinking as an adolescent rite of passage in the United States:* Drinking, and particularly binge drinking, has been widely reported as a rite of passage for adolescents in the United States (NIH 2010). It is of course potentially very dangerous; it can lead to injury, fatalities while driving, vulnerability to rape and sexual violence, severe alcohol poisoning (requiring emergency care), and more. The adolescents involved, however, are not thinking about the risk, but about doing what is perceived necessary to gain social approval in an immediate context, an imperative recognized by many psychologists (see Erikson 1963). For an adolescent, in fact, the risk of losing such approval may be viewed as a much more immediate risk than the potential and more uncertain physical and emotional costs.

- *Head hunting among the Ilongot of the Philippines:* In the past, the Ilongot people had a custom of taking a head when a loved one died. Though the practice was outlawed by the time anthropologist Renato Rosaldo and his wife, Michelle, lived among the Ilongot in the 1970s to conduct ethnographic research (Rosaldo, R. 1993, 1980; Rosaldo, M. 1980), older men still talked about the custom. It was said that Ilongot took a head because of the rage associated with grief when a loved one died. Younger men even anticipated the time that they would take their first head as a rite of passage. Rosaldo could not understand head hunting and had a hard time accepting it on moral grounds, however much he tried. It was only when his wife died in an accidental fall that he felt the kind of rage and sorrow the men talked about (though he still could not conceive of head hunting because of that). It provided a window that enabled him to at least grasp the Ilongot interpretation and to understand that his framework for understanding the act, its meaning, and its consequences was very different from theirs.

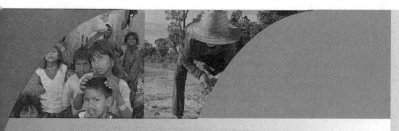

QUESTIONS

1. Think about the idea of relative risk. Are there any less-than-healthy behaviors that you have engaged in because of something you thought was more important?

2. Risk is not an absolute term; there are issues of meaning involved. How does this intersect with culture?

3. Some of the health risk behaviors described in this chapter are or were viewed as sacrifices necessary to maintain a connection with a social group. Why do you think this is such a compelling motive?

REFERENCES

Andersen, M., and M. Jenkins. 2003. *Dance of Days: Two Decades of Punk in the Nation's Capital.* New York: Akashic Books.

Cohen, M., M. Edberg, and S. Gies. 2010. *Final Report on the Evaluation of the SAGE Project.* Bethesda, MD: Development Services Group, Inc.

Douglas, M. 1992. *Risk and Blame: Essays in Cultural Theory.* London: Routledge.

Douglas, M., and A. Wildavsky. 1982. *Risk and Culture: An Essay on the Selection of Technological and Environmental Dangers.* Berkeley: University of California Press.

Edberg, M. 1994. "HIV/AIDS Risk Behavior among Runaways in the Washington, DC Metropolitan Area." In *Runaways and HIV/AIDS.* Report for National Institute on Drug Abuse (NIDA), Rockville, MD: NIDA.

Edberg, M. 2007. *Essentials of Health Behavior: Social and Behavioral Theory in Public Health.* Boston: Jones and Bartlett.

Erikson, E.H. 1963. *Childhood and Society,* 2nd ed. New York: Norton.

National Institutes of Health. 2010, October. *Underage Drinking.* Fact sheet, http://report.nih.gov/nihfactsheets/ViewFactSheet.aspx?csid=21.

Rosaldo, M.Z. 1980. *Knowledge and Passion: Ilongot Notions of Self and Social Life.* Cambridge: Cambridge University Press.

Rosaldo, R. 1980. *Ilongot Headhunting, 1883–1974: A Study in Society and History.* Palo Alto, CA: Stanford University Press.

Rosaldo, R. 1993. "Introduction: Grief and a Headhunter's Rage." In R. Rosaldo, *Culture and Truth,* (1–21). Boston, MA: Beacon Press.

Tansey, J., and T. O'Riordan. 1999. "Cultural Theory and Risk: A Review." *Health, Risk and Society* 1 (1): 71–90.

Turner, V. 1969. *The Ritual Process: Structure and Anti-Structure.* Chicago: Aldine.

Van Gennep, A. 1909 (1960). *The Rites of Passage.* London: Routledge and Kegan Paul.

World Health Organization. 2010. *Female Genital Mutilation.* Fact sheet No. 241, www.who.int/mediacentre/factsheets/fs241/en/.

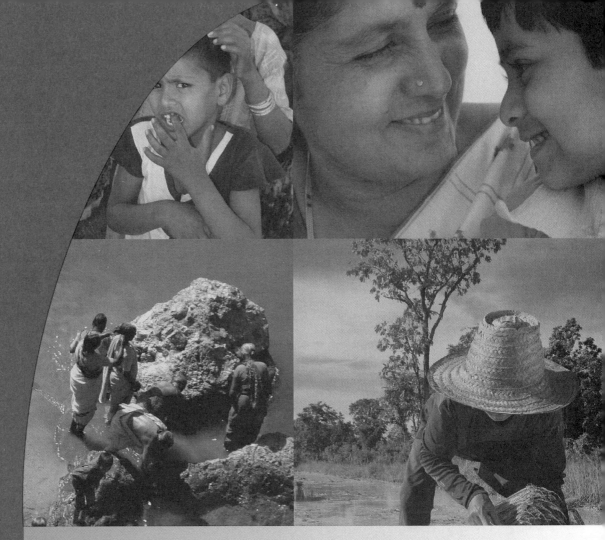

SECTION THREE

Applying Concepts of Cultural Diversity to Health Promotion

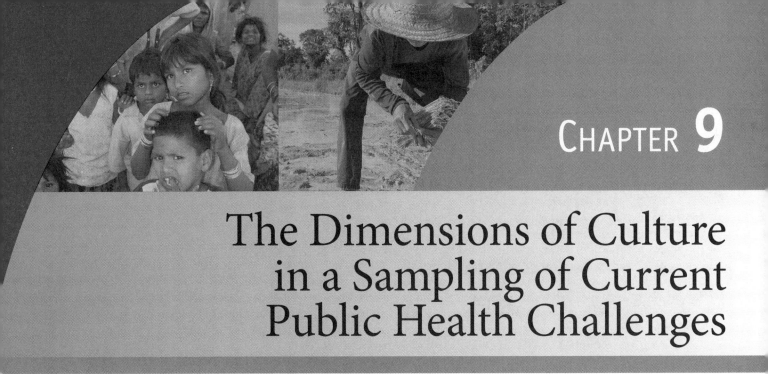

CHAPTER 9

The Dimensions of Culture in a Sampling of Current Public Health Challenges

"The body is thus not simply an 'entity,' but is experienced as a practical mode of coping with external situations and events."

—Urban anthropologist Anthony Giddens (in *Modernity and Self-Identity: Self and Society in the Late Modern Age*, 1991)

Now that you have an introductory understanding of the multiple levels at which culture has an impact on health, it will be useful to take just three examples of current and ongoing health issues and "play them out" in multiple cultural dimensions as relevant. Because they are good examples to work with, let's do this with HIV/AIDS, obesity/diabetes, and a relative newcomer to public health—youth violence. For each, we will use the tools we have gone through thus far to take a look at the key intersections of culture and health.

It's a lot to take on, but we are going to do it.

HIV/AIDS: A GRAND CANYON OF CULTURAL STRATA

The basics around HIV/AIDS were already covered in Chapter 5, so we won't repeat that information. Let's begin with the way in which different peoples think of causation for AIDS. Since 1983, biomedical research identified the virus that destroys T cells, resulting in a progressively increased vulnerability to opportunistic infection, which is the cause of mortality. By now, most people have accepted that as the single cause. But that was not always true, and it still is not always true, or, it is partially true—as when the virus as direct cause is accepted, but divine retribution for immorality or a spiritual cause is seen as behind the action of the virus.

OBESITY/DIABETES: IF WE WERE JUST HUNTER-GATHERERS AGAIN!

Obesity has become an important public health issue in the United States and globally because of its consequences—it is a major risk factor for cardiovascular disease, certain types of cancer, and type 2 diabetes (Centers for Disease Control 2011). Being obese is defined as having a body mass index (BMI) of 30 or more, calculated as a measure of weight and height; overweight is defined as a BMI between 25 and 29, with some qualifications (see Box 9-1).

Since the early 1990s, there has been a significant increase in obesity rates. In the United States by state, the data are very interesting and show important culture, lifestyle and socioeconomic differences. According to 2009 data from CDC (ibid.), only Colorado and the District of Columbia had a prevalence of obesity less than 20%! That means in every other state, at least one fifth (if not more) of the population was obese. Thirty-three states had a prevalence of 25% or more, and nine

CASE 9-1

Gender, Sexuality, and HIV/AIDS Risk in India

Addressing HIV/AIDS risk behavior in India is complicated by a number of ethnomedical beliefs, cultural traditions, and even the types of work available in the current economic situation. According to one study (Battacharya 2004), 84% of AIDS cases (at the time of the article) in India were attributed to sexual transmission. While specific population subgroups were initially at high risk, it has increasingly spread to the general population. India is highly diverse, with Hindu, Muslim, Christian, and Sikh populations. Still, a number of cultural traditions and ethnomedical beliefs cut across these lines, including:

- *Gender and family structure:* Patriarchal family structure is common, where the family name and inheritance go through the male line, from father to son. After marriage, a woman lives with her husband in her father's house. Because of the patriarchal structure, and because family wealth and resources are generally inherited by males, women find it difficult to leave marriage even if there is abuse or if the husband has extramarital sex.
- *Gender roles and ideals related to marriage:* Female purity before marriage is a prized quality, while men are encouraged to have premarital sex. Marriages are often still arranged for women near the time they reach puberty, even though the legal age of marriage for women is 18. In terms of HIV risk, men are more likely to be infected prior to marriage. If women enter marriage with knowledge about HIV risk and preventive methods, they may be suspected of having premarital sex. In addition, the female duty to procreate conflicts with condom use, and female social position is often related to childbearing, putting pressure on women not to request condom use. Condom use is also associated with sex workers—it is stigmatized. Sterilization is more common as a contraceptive than condom use. Women are sometimes sterilized when their families are completed.
- *Ethnomedical beliefs:* Commonly shared beliefs include concepts of health and balance related to flow of body fluids and regulation of heat. Condoms are sometimes viewed as interrupting this flow and thereby threatening male health. According to Battacharya's research, women may believe that their husbands are better off going to sex workers when on the road than having lovers, so that their flow is maintained without a threat to the relationship. There are also strong cultural beliefs that the marriage relationship itself is a protection from HIV/AIDS, that a woman cannot get HIV from her husband.
- *Religious traditions:* A certain acceptance of fate as part of Karma may increase acceptance of risk situations.
- *Other social patterns:* In cases of men having sex with men, it often involves men who are otherwise married.

Adding to cultural and ethnomedical factors, there is a considerable amount of migrant labor in India, a result of its rapid economic expansion. The migrant labor patterns have been internal and external—the former including rural–urban migration, and extensive work in trucking. These work contexts often mean extended periods of separation between husbands and wives and greater likelihood of casual and riskier sexual relationships.

CASE 9-2

South African Traditional Belief Systems and the Effectiveness of HIV/AIDS Prevention

Reduction of HIV/AIDS infection has remained difficult in sub-Saharan Africa. According to van Dyk (2001), the diversity of cultural groups in Africa, including those that have more Western ethnomedical beliefs, share to one degree or another a cultural worldview regarding illness/disease and sexuality (Gyeke 1987). This general set of beliefs has been at odds with most of the HIV prevention messages originating from a biomedical perspective. "Western-based education and prevention programs will therefore never succeed if the diverse cultural and belief systems in Africa are not understood and integrated into such programs" (van Dyk 2001, 61).

The generalized belief system is holistic and even human centered. It can be explained (Sow 1980) through three cosmic orders that exist within the whole: the macrocosmos, mesocosmos, and the microcosmos. They are described as follows:

- *Macrocosmos:* This consists of God, the ancestors, and the spirits of the chosen dead. However, in this system, God does not play a key role because he withdrew from human beings and left them to fend for themselves. Therefore, in this macro system, ancestors and the spirits are most important. Ancestor spirits are part of daily life for many Africans—they are usually benevolent, but they can cause harm when important social norms are violated, cultural ties are neglected, or their advice is ignored. Restoring balance with the ancestors is a necessary remedy. Typically, causality with respect to HIV/AIDS does not come from the macrocosmos, from God, or ancestors. Van Dyk (ibid.) notes that the presence of Christianity has influenced the traditional worldview for some peoples and that attributing HIV/AIDS to divine punishment is a result of such influence.

- *Mesocosmos:* This is the most important level for illness/disease causation. The mesocosmos is the dwelling place of genies, evil spirits, witches, and sorcerers. "The day-today psychological fate of individual human beings in Africa is regulated and controlled by the complex relations between humans and the invisible but powerful creatures of the meso-cosmos" (ibid., 63). With respect to illness causation, most Africans accept biomedical explanations and can hold concurrent beliefs in which, for example, infection by a pathogen is seen as an immediate cause of whatever ailment they are experiencing. At the same time, the ultimate cause—the reason behind their infection—will be understood as sorcery, witchcraft, and other machinations of the mesocosmos. Because of this, Africans may go to biomedical practitioners to treat symptoms, but may then also go to indigenous healers to identify the ultimate cause, the reason the infection came their way in the first place. HIV/AIDS is still often seen as ultimately caused by sorcery/witchcraft, particularly among individuals with less educational background, because it represents an untimely or unnatural death, which means that some spirit-level intervention occurred.

  For HIV/AIDS Prevention: Interestingly, belief in witchcraft may result in less stigma for HIV/AIDS victims because they are not blamed for their condition; at the same time, individual behavior may be viewed as less responsible. In terms of HIV/AIDS education, understanding the concurrence of witchcraft/sorcery and biomedical beliefs can be useful. The ultimate mesosystemic cause does not need to be challenged. HIV prevention information can be presented as related to the immediate cause. In addition, because various kinds of charms are understood to ward of the influence of witchcraft and sorcery, condoms could be positioned as a kind of charm.

- *Microcosmos:* This is the everyday, practical world of social relations and collective life. There are implications for HIV/AIDS causation in this realm—it is here where causation beliefs related to pollution and germs are situated. Certain ritual prohibitions against sex during menstruation, for example, are related to concepts of purity and pollution. And, even in traditional African ethnomedical systems, some diseases (e.g., colds, influenza, diarrhea, sexually transmitted infections, and malaria) are understood as caused by germs (pathogens).

  For HIV/AIDS Prevention: HIV prevention messages, as outlined by Green, Jurg, and Dgedge (1993) can be framed using traditional germ and pollution constructs. The latency period for HIV can also be translated as the *khoma* (invisible disease-causing agent, like a pathogen) hiding in the body until ready to strike. Abstention from sex while undergoing sexually transmitted disease treatment is often explained by African traditional healers in terms of avoiding pollution, yet this and similar proscriptions make for appropriate HIV prevention advice.

Finally, Van Dyk (ibid.) argues that traditional African views on sexuality link sex and children as connected to personal immortality in the mesocosmos. If a person has no offspring who remember him/her by name, when that person becomes an ancestor spirit he/she will fade into the past, no longer a member of the active spirit world. In a more practical sense (microcosmos), children represent wealth and the continuity of the family or tribe. Any HIV/AIDS messages must take this into account. At the same time, other related customs, including polygamy, may be protective against HIV infection because if faithfulness is maintained, casual sex is limited.

While most of this approach towards understanding better strategies for HIV/AIDS prevention messages focuses on ethnomedical beliefs and the incorporation of these beliefs into messaging, there is an underlying political economic issue in the argument. Essentially, the argument is that Western HIV prevention organizations and programs have come in to Africa and sought to conduct HIV/AIDS prevention based on Western beliefs and norms. It is a kind of neocolonial imposition from this point of view. Instead, indigenous beliefs and cultural systems should be recognized as legitimate and useful for HIV prevention as well.

CASE 9-3

On HIV/AIDS and Conspiracy

The author was engaged in research as part of a project to identify issues and barriers affecting the willingness of injection drug and crack users to come and get HIV tested at public or community clinics in Washington, DC (the project was funded by a small grant from the National Institute on Drug Abuse in the mid-1990s). The goal was to use this information to train public clinic staff, to improve their capabilities to work with this subpopulation, and to design a communications approach that would increase HIV testing.

A number of focus groups were conducted with a sample of the population, in mobile vans/recreational vehicles already being used for outreach and other programs in the city. In addition to widely reported experiences of stigma and manifestly negative attitudes (from staff) at these clinics, two other themes repeatedly arose:

1. HIV/AIDS, like drug abuse, was seen as prevalent in the community because of either a conspiracy to do harm to African Americans or a negligent willingness to let the problem fester without providing any help or support. Beliefs about the causes of HIV/AIDS were therefore situated within broader beliefs about, and experiences of, racism and generally malicious intentions from the dominant white population.

2. There was a deep mistrust about providing blood to a public clinic, explicitly tied in focus group comments to the infamous Tuskegee experiments conducted by the U.S. Public Health Service and Tuskegee Institute (Alabama) from 1932 to 1972, in which poor, rural black men were enlisted in an experiment to study the natural progression of syphilis. In that experiment, the men regularly gave blood as part of their participation and were never told they had syphilis and never offered treatment for it. Even though the study had ended many years before, and revelations about its ethical lapses contributed to what are now extensive protections for human subjects involved in research, the magnitude of the deception was still contributing to the mistrust about public health institutions widely shared in this drug user population.

As a result of this information, project results included a recommendation and a strategy to build a communications approach that acknowledged these beliefs and experiences. The idea was to use a "knowledge-is-power" theme—that is, knowledge of HIV status—in connection with a call to fight the "conspiracy" of HIV/AIDS.

FIGURE 9-1 Why HIV/AIDS?

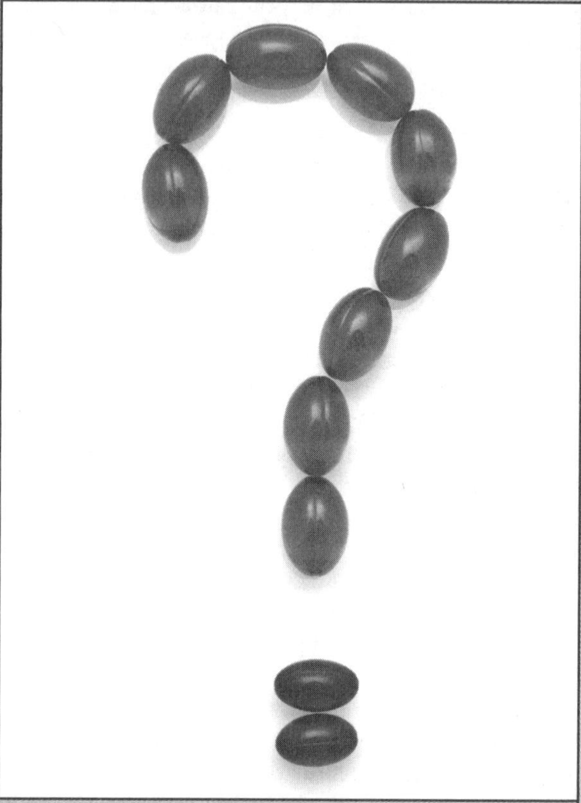

Source: © drkaczmar/ShutterStock, Inc.

BOX 9-1 Definitions of Overweight and Obesity for Adults

For adults, overweight and obesity ranges are determined by using weight and height to calculate a number called the "body mass index." BMI is used because, for most people, it correlates with their amount of body fat.

- An adult who has a BMI between 25 and 29.9 is considered overweight.
- An adult who has a BMI of 30 or higher is considered obese.

Table 9-1 provides examples for a person who is 5 feet, 9 inches tall.

TABLE 9-1 BMI

Height	Weight range	BMI	Considered
5'9"	124 lbs or less	Below 18.5	Underweight
	125 lbs to 168 lbs	18.5 to 24.9	Healthy weight
	169 lbs to 202 lbs	25.0 to 29.9	Overweight
	203 lbs or more	30 or higher	Obese

It is important to remember that although BMI correlates with the amount of body fat, BMI does not directly measure body fat. As a result, some people (e.g., athletes), who have a lot of muscle, may have a BMI that falls in the category of overweight even though they do not have excess body fat.

Other methods of estimating body fat and body fat distribution include measurements of skinfold thickness and waist circumference, calculation of waist-to-hip circumference ratios, and techniques such as ultrasound, computed tomography, and magnetic resonance imaging.

Definitions for Children and Adolescents

For children and adolescents, BMI ranges above a normal weight have different labels (overweight and obese). Additionally, BMI ranges for children and adolescents are defined so that they take into account normal differences in body fat between boys and girls and differences in body fat at various ages.

Source: From U.S. Centers for Disease Control and Prevention 2011.

of these states (Alabama, Arkansas, Kentucky, Louisiana, Mississippi, Missouri, Oklahoma, Tennessee, and West Virginia) had a prevalence of obesity equal to or greater than 30%. A few other statistics fill in the story: Obesity rates are highest for African Americans at 35.7% overall, followed by Hispanic Americans at 28.7%, then by white, non-Hispanics at 23.7%. This is a serious issue. Take a look at Figure 9-2, which shows obesity by state (percentages below the figure refer to BMI).

Globally, the situation is similar. The World Health organization (WHO) estimated that in 2008, approximately 1.5 billion adults (age 20 or older) were overweight, and of these, 200 million men and almost 300 million women were obese (WHO 2011). They also project that by 2015, 2.3 billion adults will be overweight and 700 million will be obese.

Yet hunger is still a serious global problem, affecting some 780 million people in developing countries and 815 million overall, according to the United Nations Food and Agriculture Organization (2002). But even a decade ago, the Worldwatch Institute (Gardner & Halweil 2000) released data showing that, for the first time, the number of overweight individuals worldwide rivals those who are underweight. In addition to China, many developing economies are experiencing fast-growing rates of obesity. In Brazil and Columbia, some 40% of people

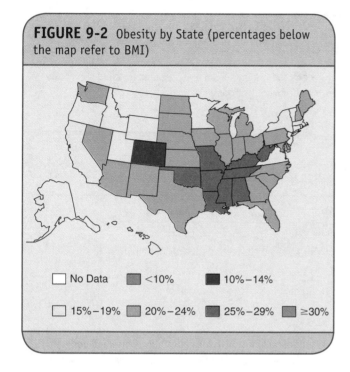

FIGURE 9-2 Obesity by State (percentages below the map refer to BMI)

No Data   <10%   10%–14%

15%–19%   20%–24%   25%–29%   ≥30%

forms of work, changing modes of transportation, and increasing urbanization. (WHO 2011: 2)

A more specific list, with an orientation to causes in the United States, includes the following (French, Story, and Jeffery 2001; Jeffery and Utter, 2003):

- Extensive marketing of unhealthy food products (including fast food)
- Overeating
- Lack of exercise
- Increased reliance on vehicle transportation
- A sedentary lifestyle related in part to the ubiquity of television, computers, and other labor-saving technologies
- Changes in the quality of available foods
- Increased portion sizes
- Trends towards eating out
- The growth of the convenience food industry
- Increased advertising by the food industry

Let's break out some of these issues by relevant dimensions of cultural influence.

Obesity and Cultural Factors

It is important to acknowledge that until very recently, obesity was not viewed by most people in the world as a disease or illness. Treating it in that way is new. So in ethnomedical terms, you might not find it on the list of "states of being unwell." The diseases with which it is associated, such as diabetes and cardiovascular disease, on the other hand, are likely to be on those lists. So, its ethnomedical location is somewhat complicated. To add another complication, knowledge about the connections between overweight/obesity and those health conditions may or may not be widespread. If not, it won't be part of the ethnomedical picture.

Some of the most important behavioral causes of obesity—diet and eating practices—are culturally very thick. There is a lot bound up in what we eat and how we eat. The elements of a good meal are culturally generated and are part of what it means to live a good life or live well. Typically, cultural diets also include foods that are thought of as curative, like the stereotypical chicken soup. And food is very much tied to identity—Italians

were overweight, according to the Food and Agriculture Organization (FAO). This rate is similar to European countries. Even in sub-Saharan Africa (where hunger is a widespread problem), there has been an increase in obesity, especially among urban women. Interestingly, globalization has changed the face of obesity according to the FAO. Where overweight used to be a sign of wealth, it is now becoming a sign of poverty. Those who are wealthier have more access to the tools of healthy lifestyles, including exercise facilities (and the time to use them), and better foods.

A Preventable Condition. When it comes to culture and its influence, here is the key point regarding obesity: It is an entirely preventable condition, the prevalence of which is almost entirely related to patterns of diet and exercise—in turn, powerfully influenced by any and all of the elements of cultural influence discussed in this book. As summarized by WHO (2011), obesity and overweight are caused by:

1) a global shift in diet towards increased intake of energy-dense foods that are high in fat and sugars but low in vitamins, minerals and other micronutrients; and 2) a trend towards decreased physical activity due to the increasingly sedentary nature of many

swear by good Italian food just like Ghanaians swear by good Ghanaian food. These connections are also complex in themselves; conceptions of what constitutes food or a meal, as well as how foods should be consumed and prepared, vary by ethnicity, geographic region, gender, age, and social class (Pollock 1992; Reid 1986; Weismantel 1988). How meals are eaten and the social behavior involved is yet another important cultural layer. Food sharing is commonly associated with strong individual, family, and group ties and often invokes values of hospitality, mutual caring, group solidarity, and common goals, as well as social and even political obligations. When an ambassador holds a state dinner, you can be sure that the details of the food to be served and how it is served have been carefully planned. Or, you may have been in situations yourself where you were having dinner with a family from a different culture, and found that they paid a lot of attention to your willingness to eat their food, and your enjoyment (or not) of that food! Showing that willingness is a signal and may provide your first cultural entrée.

If it is future in-laws with whom you are eating, that signal may carry a lot of weight. It may be (on a light note) a case of relative risk—in that situation, refusing to eat food even if you think it's not healthy might constitute a risk!

There is an important political-economic dimension to diet. Access to healthy food is related to class and social inequities. In the United States, numerous studies have documented the lack of supermarkets, farmers' markets, and grocery stores in low-income areas (e.g., Weinberg 2000; Morland et al. 2001). These kinds of stores are more likely to have fresh fruits and vegetables. In other words, choice of food is limited by where one lives in some cases, and that is related to a socioeconomic status.

Another behavioral cause of obesity is the lack of physical exercise, which is connected to cultural practices and beliefs, and to political-economic factors. Most of the world does not think of exercise as a leisure activity that one does apart from work. Physical exertion is part of the kinds of work many people do, from farm work, to construction work, to the day-to-day labors of getting water and firewood. In that sense, it is integrated into cultural patterns of daily life, which are themselves related to social class and occupational opportunity (a political-economic factor). It is primarily in wealthy and industrialized economies or white-collar job sectors where the idea of going to exercise means something people do after or in between work. After all, that kind of exercise is usually connected to a place or a facility—like a track, or a health club, or a gym. One qualification: there is also a distinction to be made between exercise in that sense and sport. Playing a sport as recreation involves exercise, but again, if you think about young people playing soccer in a Brazilian *favela*, for example, the attraction is probably to the sport, the competition, and friends, much more than an abstract idea of exercise.

While restrictions on healthy diet and exercise are most often characteristic of urban, high-poverty communities, rural poverty has a similar effect. West Virginia has the highest rate of obesity among white, non-Hispanics at just over 30% obese and another 38% overweight. In data collected by the U.S. Centers for Disease Control and Prevention, almost 30% of West Virginians reported no leisure-time physical activity in the past month, and only 1 in 5 adults eat fruits and vegetables five or more times a day. And in 2008, almost 18% of the state's population lived below the poverty line (U.S. Census Bureau 2009).

There is another very important political-economic factor connected to exercise. As economies become more globalized and industrialized, a lot of the work is sedentary, in front of a computer or technical device of some kind. A lot of play activity is also sedentary, involving sitting at a computer or in front of a TV or increasingly involving cell phones and tablet computers. Yet another political-economic factor is that people living in urban areas of dense poverty and with high rates of crime can't just go out and jog around the park, and neither can their children. This can accentuate the use of sedentary technology as recreation.

Another cultural influence is body size and what it means. Not everyone subscribes to the Western thin look. For some peoples, having a large body size is synonymous with being well or at least living well, which in itself could signify a person of status or in some cases royalty. Being thin may signify poverty, starvation, not living well, and lower status (see Douglas & Wildavsky 1982). There is also a gender factor for body size. It is interesting to see that in the United States, obesity rates are higher for women than men except among white non-Hispanics. Larger body size is more normative for African American and Latina women than it is for non-Hispanic, white women. This is mediated by region—obesity rates are higher for all categories in the South and Midwest, which is a reflection of diet and exercise patterns.

BOX 9-2 A Current Issue: Diet, Obesity, and Immigrant/Refugee Populations

Immigrants to the United States often enter in better health than the average American (Singh & Miller 2004). Eventually, however, the health status of these immigrants often declines over time. Part of this change has to do with diet. When immigrants become acculturated to diet patterns in the United States, it can have detrimental effects on health. Many studies have looked at immigrant populations in the United States—particularly Latinos—and found clear connections between acculturation and obesity (Kaiser Family Foundation 2005). Diet acculturation, though, is accompanied by other issues, such as:

- Working many jobs; no leisure or exercise time
- Exercise as a discrete activity not necessarily being a cultural pattern
- Living in neighborhoods without access to safe parks or recreation areas
- Technology change, television etc., and the reduction of community and neighbor interaction compared to their home country situation
- Using and having high-tech commodities (flat-screen televisions, computers, video games, etc.) as symbols of success—leading to reduced physical activity
- Use of vehicles—reduction of walking compared to home country pattern
- Food change—increase in fast food (possibly seen as a sign of success), decrease in local natural food

When migrants arrive in a country where food is less scarce, more likely to be processed as well as higher in sugar, fats, and carbohydrates, and at the same time they enter at low levels of socioeconomic status, a pattern of obesity may ensue (and has been documented—see, for example, Sundquist & Wikelby 2000; Khan, Sobal, & Martorell 1997). For some populations, the prestige attached to being large as a signifier of wealth and well-being may be retained (see, for example, Renzaho 2004) and contribute to obesity.

Cultural Ecology: The Hunter-Gatherer Diet and Contemporary Living Patterns

The kind of diets often touted by doctors and nutritionists as ideal, like the Mediterranean diet or other diets rich in fruits, nuts, beans, vegetables, and grains, with a limited amount of meat (especially red meat), is a lot like the diet eaten by earlier human cultures who were not yet settled in cities or states.[1] They hunted, with just occasional success, and spent a lot of time gathering available plant foods and fruit—hence the name hunter-gatherer. As far as we know, they did not have any problem with overweight or obesity. They were not eating foods high in sugar or fat, and the human metabolism was adapted to the diet pattern (Eaton, Shostak, & Konner 1988).

At the same time, food shortages from time to time were not abnormal. For that reason, humans had a mechanism for storing energy as fat. This may have had a gender dimension that resonates today. There is evidence of an association between fat and fertility in women, which may relate to greater energy reserves and the ability to withstand food shortages (Brown & Konner 1987). Many cultures have rituals where girls reaching puberty are urged to "fatten up"; plumpness (but not obesity) is rated as a desirable female characteristic in 81% of societies for which there are data (ibid.—cross-cultural comparisons from the Human Relations Area Files). The propensity for obesity also differs naturally by gender—in almost all human populations, females have more body fat than males. Typically this is called peripheral or limb fat, which is not associated with many of the diseases of obesity (type 2 diabetes or hypertension). Trunk or centripetal fat is. Women remain more susceptible than men to obesity (ibid.).

YOUTH VIOLENCE: SERIOUS ENOUGH FOR PUBLIC HEALTH

Youth violence is relatively new on the public health agenda, but because it is such a leading cause of mortality and morbidity for young people—young men in particular—it has become a significant issue. According to the World Health Organization, violence is "one of

---

[1] Of course there was variation in this diet, depending upon where people lived and what kinds of foods were available.

CASE 9-4

Emerging Obesity in China

According to one summary of data from a 2002 national study of health and nutrition in China (see Markey 2006), 15% of adults in China (about 200 million Chinese) are overweight. Of these, 7% (90 million) are obese (by contrast: 30% of U.S. adults are obese). The problem in China has begun to affect children and youth. Since about 2000, China's childhood obesity rate has doubled. The problem is worst in urban areas.

The same study indicated that almost 17% of urban school-age boys and almost 10% of school-age girls were obese in China. The average Chinese 6-year-old is now very similar in weight and height to his/her American counterparts. The causes are not mysterious. They include:

- Diets of Chinese adults and children are far higher in calorie-heavy meats, fish, eggs, dairy products, fats and sugars than they were for many years prior to the study.
- Children/youth are sedentary today, spending much more time indoors in front of homework, television, computer games, and the Internet.
- Many Chinese youth have pocket money and spend a lot of it on junk food—which bring prestige, fed by advertising and peer norms.

McDonald's, Kentucky Fried Chicken, and other American fast-food companies now have hundreds of outlets in China. Auto sales have tripled since 2006. Yet only 45 years ago, during the Cultural Revolution, China was in the midst of a serious famine. Some 30 million people died of starvation. Even today, there is malnourishment and starvation in rural areas—24 million Chinese suffer from malnutrition. Bigger children may still be a source of pride and proof of prosperity for many Chinese. The change in China's experience with obesity and its consequences has occurred since about 2000, much faster than it happened in the Western developed countries, and very much in line with China's rapid economic growth—a clear political-economic aspect of the issue.

Chinese adults between age 35 and 64 are now twice as likely to die of heart disease than Americans of the same age, according to WHO. There has also been a dramatic increase in surgeries to treat weight-related illnesses.

the leading public health issues of our time" (Krug et al., 2002), particularly youth violence. Violence irrespective of age category is among the main causes of death for people aged 15–44 years of age, yet interpersonal violence among young adults aged 15–29 was responsible for 36.2% of that total (ibid.). Despite some indications of a downturn in U.S. rates for youth violence during 2007–2008, serious violent crimes by youth and young adults have continued to rise. Moreover, "national rates also mask variation among cities, many of which report ongoing increases in perpetration of violent crime and weapons offenses by this age group during the first two quarters of 2010" (Browne et al. 2010: 56). The increases are typically in selected high-poverty communities and related to youth/young adults under age 25 (Butts & Snyder 2006). Intentional violence is the leading cause of

death for African American youth age 10–24, the second leading cause of death for Latino youth, and the third leading cause for Asian/Pacific Islander and American Indian/Alaska Native youth (CDC 2010). In general, homicide was the second leading cause of death for young people 10–24 years old in 2007, and 84% of those victims were killed with a firearm (ibid.). Moreover, while the homicide rate in 2007 for Hispanic males was more than 5 times the rate for Caucasian males, the rate for African American youth was about 3 times the Hispanic rate (and more than 15 times the Caucasian rate). In short, it is an ongoing and serious national issue.

What is the role of culture? In the case of youth violence, the cultural role is heavily conditioned by structural factors—that is, political economy. This is one of those situations where, as described in Chapter 8, the

CASE 9-5

Obesity and Type 2 Diabetes among Pima Indians: The Impact of Cultural Ecology on Disease

The Pima Indians (the real tribal name is Akimel O'odham—they are related to other O'odham peoples in the area) are believed to have lived for over 2,000 years in the valleys of the Gila and Salt Rivers—which is located in modern-day Arizona. They are likely descendants of the ancient Hohokam people. For centuries, the Pimas' way of life was sustained by irrigation farming accompanied by hunting and gathering food. Then came a dramatic change in political-economic circumstances, which had a great impact on Pima health. From the late 17th century, the Spanish and Mexican presence was influential. Following the Mexican-American War and then the Gadsden Purchase of 1853, the territory came under American control and there was a migration of settlers moving west, resulting in a dramatic change for the Pima. By the late 19th century, the traditional way of life was disrupted by settlers, and the Pima were moved to reservation land.

Importantly, much of the traditional diet was eliminated because settlers essentially cut off the Pimas' water supply by building dams. The Gila River, source of irrigation for crops and fish for food, is now dry (though some water has been restored to Pima lands following a long legal battle and the concluding of the Arizona Water Settlement in 2004, providing water from other area dams—see Brown 2009). The nearby Salt and Verde Rivers were also interrupted by dams and subsequently became dry. This caused a dramatic change in culture and lifestyle for the Pimas. The Pimas came to rely on lard, sugar, and flour provided by the U.S. government to survive. Previously, a traditional Pima diet was high in starch and fiber and only contained about 15% fat. Key foods included cholla cactus buds, honey mesquite, poverty weed, and prickly pears (a cactus) from the desert floor; mule deer, white-winged dove, and black jackrabbit; squawfish from the Gila River; and wheat, squash, and beans grown in irrigated desert fields. Today, 40% of the calories in the Pima diet are obtained from fat (NIDDK 2009).

Obesity and its consequences have been for some time a significant problem for the Pimas (Knowler et al. 1991). Over 50% of Pima adults have type 2 diabetes, and 95% of these individuals with diabetes are overweight (ibid.). Data show that Pimas are much heavier now than those at the beginning of the century, and weights have continued to increase. Young children and adults are particularly affected by this epidemic. A study comparing Pimas who lived in Mexico versus those who lived in Arizona found that while genetically similar, Mexican Pimas had very low rates of diabetes and were generally not overweight. This is attributed to a higher level of physical activity as well as a diet with less fat among Mexican Pimas.

Studies have also found that obesity in Pimas is familial (see for example, Knowler et al. 1991). An example of this can be seen in Pima women who are pregnant—if a pregnant woman is diabetic (and most likely overweight)—this leads to early onset of diabetes and obesity in the child. The genetic connection may be related to a biocultural phenomenon called the "thrifty gene syndrome": Peoples like the Pimas who lived for thousands of years on traditional foods that may have varied dramatically in availability due to climate evolved a thrifty gene allowing individuals to store fat when food was available to prevent starvation when food was scarce. However, with a change in diet to high-caloric diet, this genetic characteristic is maladaptive.

Traditional Culture. Traditionally, the Pima lived in villages of domed brush roundhouses. Pima women produced cotton fabric and made intricately woven watertight basketry, patterned with black and white. A council of elders and a hereditary chief governed village affairs by consensus, and land was farmed cooperatively. Much of the Pima's traditional culture and way of life has now been lost; most Pima have been Catholic since the 18th century due to the impact of Spanish missionaries and control of the territory until the 1800s. However, traditional religions/ceremonies (according to earlier ethnographies and descriptions) included the rain ceremony, harvest dance, and the war dance (the latter involved the ceremonial use of scalps). Puberty rites, called the "changing," were also celebrated by the Pima. The Pima creation myth is very complex, centering on Chuwutumaka (earth doctor), the creator.

CASE 9-6

Obesity and Type 2 Diabetes among Samoans: Traditional Ideas of the Body and the Impact of Western Diets

Once again, we have a case example that is in part the result of political-economic history influencing cultural patterns. Samoans are a major Pacific Islander culture group, related to other Pacific Islander peoples, including Native Hawaiians. The Samoan Islands are in the South Pacific, between New Zealand and Hawaii, and are split between the western and eastern groups of islands. Samoans are Polynesians, and early settlers to Samoa came from other Southeast Asia and Melanesia. Western influence began with a Dutch explorer, soon followed by others, including missionaries. In the mid-19th century, British, German, and American interests were competing for control. A treaty was signed at the turn of the 20th century, partitioning Samoa into American (eastern) and German (western) islands. During World War I, New Zealand took control over German territories and retained this under League of Nations mandate until these islands became independent in 1962. Western and American Samoa have since diverged somewhat in socioeconomic and political patterns, with American Samoans much more likely to adopt Western/American lifestyle patterns and migrate to the United States. Then, from about the time of World War II, American Samoa became a large U.S. naval and marine base (Pago Pago Harbor), exerting a strong cultural influence.

Western influence, modernization, and—for American Samoa—migration, has had a significant impact on issues of obesity and diabetes. According to recent data, 80% of female migrants in Hawaii are overweight, compared to 46% of those who live traditionally (more so in Western Samoa). A majority of Samoans who live in Hawaii are obese by the time they reach 30 (Davis et al. 2004; McGarvey 1991).

Centuries ago, Samoans engaged in agriculture, and men would go on long sailing and fishing expeditions—it is hypothesized that the Samoans (like the Pima) have a thrifty-gene phenomenon, where being able to store food energy efficiently with excess body weight was beneficial to the sailors' survival—a genetic trait passed down to subsequent generations. There is, however, no proof for this hypothesis.

Environmental influences, combined with aspects of Samoan culture, are an important factor on Samoan obesity: the lack of occupation-related physical activity, traditional Sunday feasting, access to high caloric foods (such as Spam musubi—rice blocks topped with spam and wrapped in seaweed), and traditional cultural acceptance of a robust physique (ibid.).

Among Polynesian peoples, large body size has traditionally symbolized the power and status of royal or powerful individuals, a cultural view of body type that persists to some degree today. In addition, Western fast food has come to American Samoa, with McDonald's, KFC and Pizza Hut being very popular. An interesting cultural sidelight is the role of Spam as a popular part of Samoan diet, likely as a result of American military presence in World War II. Buying imported foods such as rice is also viewed as a sign of prestige. By contrast, traditional Samoan foods were much healthier, including fish, shellfish, pork, many roots such as taro, and bananas, breadfruit, and coconuts.

Additional Traditional Cultural Elements. Traditional Samoan culture and social organization, still important today, was dominated by a structure of power closely integrated with food resources (see Bindon 2006). Villages are governed by a council or *fono* and led by a titled chief or *matai* (there are also talking chiefs). The power of the *matai* was often symbolized and underscored by his or her role in the control and distribution of food. Living arrangements were traditionally communal, in large, open houses, with little privacy. Regular (Sunday) feasting is important. Samoans are largely Christian now, but there are many traditional creation myths and legendary figures, including the existence of a spirit realm called Pulotu. Dance, tattooing, and a number of sports such as rugby (and now American football) are popular.

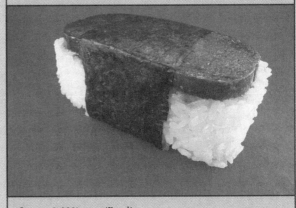

FIGURE 9-3 "Spam Musubi"—Hawaiian Dish Made with Spam

Source: © 808isgreat/Fotolia

BOX 9-3   Are Sumo Wrestlers Healthy?

To illustrate the point about culture and definitions of health, let's take the case of sumo wrestlers.

Brief Background: Sumo wrestling is an ancient Japanese martial art form that began to flourish in the Edo (or Tokugawa) period of Japanese history (from 1603 to 1867), but drew on many older traditions of court wrestling, and from Shinto religious traditions. Wrestlers are generally called *rikishi*, and bouts are fought in a circular ring known as the *dohyo*. The basics are simple—the object of the match is to force one's opponent out of the ring or to force him to touch the ground with anything other than the soles of his feet. Strength, power, and size are therefore paramount.

Most sumo wrestlers live in communal training stables called *"heya,"* in which their lives are strictly regulated by tradition, from meals to dress, as monitored and managed by the Japanese Sumo Association. According to the association, there are currently 54 training stables and a total of 700 wrestlers. The wrestlers are also organized according to a clear hierarchy by ability. From the highest level down, this is: *makuuchi* (maximum 42 wrestlers); *juryo* (fixed at 28 wrestlers); *makushita* (fixed at 120 wrestlers); *sandanme* (fixed at 200 wrestlers); *jonidan* (approximately 230 wrestlers); and *jonokuchi* (approximately 80 wrestlers). In the top 2 classes, wrestlers are called *"sekitori,"* while the rest are just referred to as *rikishi*. There is a separate hierarchy within the top *makuuchi* class. At the lower level of this class are about 16 or 17 wrestlers, in ranked order, called *maegashira*. Above them are 3 titleholder ranks, together known as *sanyaku* (from *komusubi*, *sekiwake*, up to *ozeki*). Above that is the highest sumo level, the *yokozuna*.

FIGURE 9-4 Sumo Wrestlers

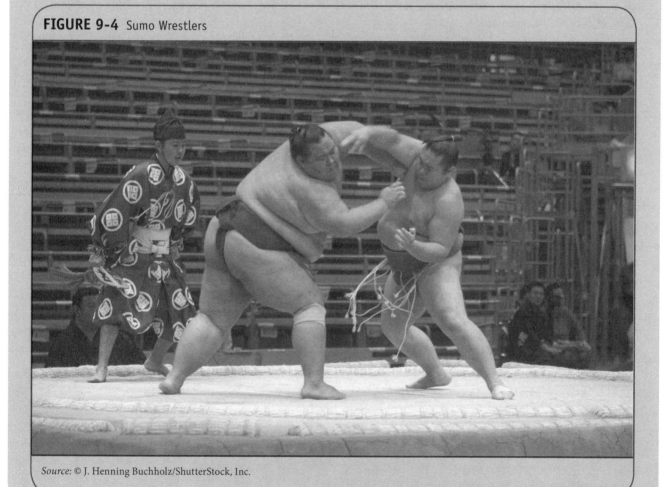

Source: © J. Henning Buchholz/ShutterStock, Inc.

BOX 9-3 *(Continued)*

On the Dietary Aspects of Their Training: Sumo wrestlers may eat as many as 8,000 kilocalories per day, more than twice that of an average Japanese adult male. A wrestler's day begins about 5 a.m. with morning training. Working out on an empty stomach helps slow down the body's metabolism and makes burning calories more difficult. At around 11 a.m., the wrestlers have their first feast of the day—*chankonabe*—the staple diet of sumo wrestlers. It is a one-pot stew, and anything can go into it. Many different meats, vegetables, and fish are cooked in the boiling chicken broth soup base. *Chankonabe* is very rich in protein and usually served in large quantities with other side dishes. Some wrestlers eat 5 kilograms of meat or 10 bowls of rice in one meal. For wrestlers who are not yet huge, gaining weight can be difficult. They will continue to gorge on large meals until they throw up—a famous part of the sumo wrestlers' harsh diet training. After eating the first meal of the day, sumo wrestlers take a long nap in the afternoon in order to help them gain weight, since the food is being stored as fat. Then they come back again to the dining table around 6 or 7 p.m.

Sources: Japanese Sumo Association (www.sumo.or.jp/eng/); CNN at http://www.cnngo.com/tokyo/none/secrets-sumo-wrestlers-diet-067161.

risk posed by violence has to be understood in terms of the contexts where violence is most prevalent, largely in urban communities of concentrated poverty.

Many of these communities are virtually disconnected from mainstream economic institutions and opportunities, and as a result have evolved underground or street economies of their own. In terms of what we have written about in the book, these economies and their accompanying social structures and subcultures are an adaptation, within a social ecology, to marginalization and limited opportunity (Wilkinson, Beaty, and Lurry 2009; Wilkinson 2004; Bourgois 1996; Wilson 1987; Sampson and Wilson 1995). One problem, though, is that these alternate or substitute economies are not formal and are typically (though not always) unstable and volatile. In the drug market, for example, there is a potential for a significant amount of money, and so many people try to get involved and to gain control. The ongoing struggle for control is usually violent, and over time, violence as a means of establishing power, demonstrating power, and asserting status becomes a community norm. For young people growing up in that environment, it may be clear that violence is part of how one becomes someone who matters. Without competing possibilities and few job paths, the risks associated with violence may be relative. Being well or doing well, in the sense that we have talked about in this book, may not be associated with a long and productive life, but with having the capability to rise to

the top of the heap and establish a reputation, even if it is for a short time. The rationale: At least for that short time you achieved some measure of respect; you mattered. A kind of subculture grows up around this situation.

This is exactly what I found in a study along the U.S. Mexican border area with respect to the attitudes of young people living in very poor *colonias* (shantytown neighborhoods), as well as people from rural areas (Edberg 2004a, 2004b) towards narcotraffickers and the violence associated with them. The violence and other exploits were featured in a popular song genre called *corridos* (traditionally, these songs were about Mexican populist heroes—when they are about narcotraffickers, they are called *narcocorridos*). Many youth interviewed for this study expressed a desire to have *corridos* written and sung about them, like those sung about popular narcotraffickers, even though the narcocorridos described violence, risk, and treachery.

Thinking about what we have discussed in terms of relative risk, narcotraffickers were positioned by these songs as individuals who stood out, who possessed something special. As noted in the report on the study:

> Risk, even risk of death, was viewed as the currency that could elevate a youth who lived in the dusty squalor of the border colonias into a kind of pantheon of the notable, to be among those who "made a dent in the

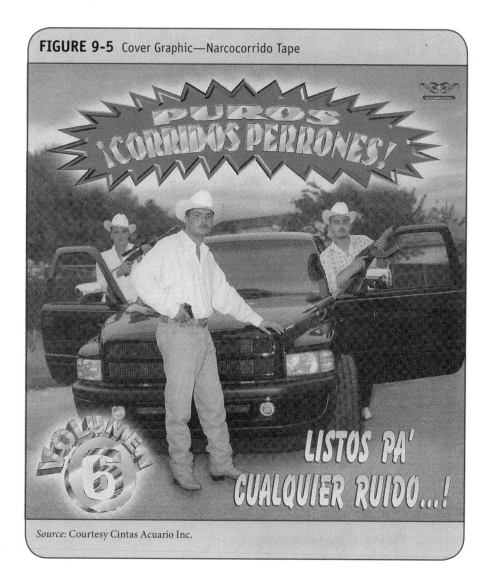

FIGURE 9-5 Cover Graphic—Narcocorrido Tape

Source: Courtesy Cintas Acuario Inc.

cosmos," so to speak, and were recognized for doing so—something that regular life in the colonias was not likely to offer. Even if the end-result was death, the attainment of any notoriety was perceived as better than the poverty, facelessness and lack of respect they expected otherwise. (Edberg and Bourgois, forthcoming).

These views are supported by a growing border area narcoculture that has its own patron "saint," a bandit-hero called Jesus Malverde, with a shrine in the Mexican city of Culiacán

This is also what other researchers have found when investigating urban street cultures where violence is prevalent, in particular identifying what Elijah Anderson called the "code of the street" (1999).

It is also something that is very much elaborated in gang culture. While definitions of what a gang is continue to be elusive, it is one of the key social formations linked to violence as well as violent beliefs and attitudes. The issue of gangs and gang culture is not new. There is a whole school of urban social research called the "Chicago School" after the many studies of urban ills—including gangs—that came out of the University of Chicago, beginning with Robert Park and publication of

BOX 9-4 Common Elements of Gang Culture

1. *Name*—Could be a street, neighborhood, a version of a larger moiety/family like *Locos, Surenos*, Crips. For Latino gangs, the number 13 may in part refer to M as the 13th letter, and it refers to *Mara* (gang) or Mexican Mafia.

2. *Organization into Structures and Substructures*—Gang clans or families such as Crips and Bloods, MS-13, and so on, have typically broken up into ever-changing cliques or sets. There may be generations involved, from older gang leaders (often called "OGs" or "original gangstas"), to younger wannabes or initiates.

3. *Origin Myths and Stories*—Institutionalized stories or myths about the origin of the gang, the origin of its symbols, and the original gang members/founders.

4. *Uniforms/Colors/Markings*—Includes specific colors, clothing elements worn specific ways, tattoos, scarring, or other marking.

5. *Physical Signs*—Hand signs, body movement/dance signs, others.

6. *Othering Processes*—These result in rivalries. New gang members learn "slur terms" for other gangs, other ways to disrespect them.

7. *Gender Roles*—There are often female auxiliaries with specific (sometimes violent) roles and connections to male gang units, or, more recently, female gangs or sets. Females may also have traditional role relationships with male gang members.

8. *Initiations*—Includes "jumping in," committing a criminal or violent act to prove capability, "baptism" or other situations. Female gang members may be "sexed in."

9. *Graffiti*—Usually with numbers, coded numbers, and terms for gang name, street, etc. For messaging and marking territory.

10. *Territory*—Sometimes, not always.

Examples of Gang Names:
- *Caucasian/White gangs:* Aryan Brotherhood, skinheads, Street Fighters, Nazi Low Riders, Hells Angels, Pagans
- *Southeast Asian gangs (Sacramento, CA examples):* Tiny Rascal Gangsters (Cambodian, Lao, Hmong, Vietnamese); Masters of Destruction (Hmong); IVB/Insane Viet Boy (Vietnamese, Viet-Chinese); Asian Pride (Many Southeast Asian groups); Asian Boyz (Vietnamese, Cambodian); GD/Green Dragon (Vietnamese); Hmong Nation Society (Hmong)
- *Latino gangs:* Latin Kings (Puerto Rican, Mexican—Chicago and New York), *Mara Salvatrucha* or MS-13 (Salvadoran, Central American), 18th Street, *Vatos Locos, Surenos, Nortenos, Locos, Maravillas*
- *African American gangs:* Crips, Bloods, Pirus, Black Guerillas, Black Peace Stone Nation, Vice Lords (Chicago). Sometimes organized into smaller, looser, neighborhood crews.
- *Native American gangs:* Wild Boyz, Indian Mafia, Nomads
- *Caribbean/Jamaican gangs:* Posses. In Jamaica, often tied to political parties (with colors).

Source: Adapted from New Jersey Office of the Attorney General N.D.:

The City in 1925, and Frederick M. Thrasher's *The Gang* in 1927. One of the most famous early anthropological studies of gangs was *Street Corner Society*, by William Foote Whyte (1993/43), about Italian gangs in the slums of Boston. In Los Angeles, James Diego Vigil (2007) has long been conducting research on generations of Mexican-American gang culture. In Europe, the issue has surfaced in the work of anthropologist Ulf Hannerz and by current work—a project called EuroGang.

Given some of the stereotypes, it is important to remember that gangs are not exclusive to ethnic minority populations, but more generally to populations that are marginalized and living in poor conditions. In the United States' urban areas, there have been Irish gangs,

Italian gangs, Chinese gangs, Jewish gangs, and many more—before the advent of the more contemporary Latino, Asian, and African American gangs. There have been biker gangs as well, at least since the 1950s (Hell's Angels), and skinhead gangs. There is even a gang subcategory called prison gangs. All have their own cultures and subcultures, some that have developed and been passed down over a long period of time.

Given these cultural (and political-economic) factors, interventions to address youth violence may usefully try to incorporate this kind of information in program design, in the same way other public health interventions do.

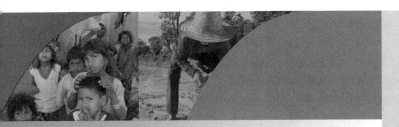

QUESTIONS

1. What link can be made between political-economic factors and the differences in approach to HIV/AIDS prevention messages discussed earlier in the chapter?

2. How would you address HIV/AIDS risk in a context where gender roles create risk, but (as in India) are deeply embedded in cultural and economic patterns?

3. In the case the Pima, the traditional diet and activity pattern was not at all conducive to obesity. What could you do in a prevention program that would incorporate that?

4. Sumo wrestlers are admired cultural icons. Do you think people think of them as obese or unhealthy?

5. What aspects of culture are at work in behaviors and attitudes about violence among youth?

REFERENCES

Anderson, E. (1999). *Violence and the Inner City Street Code.* Chicago, IL: University of Chicago Press.

Battacharya, G. 2004. "Sociocultural and Behavioral Contexts of Condom Use in Heterosexual Married Couples in India: Challenges to the HIV Prevention Program." *Health Education and Behavior* 31 (1): 101–117.

Bindon, J. "Food, Power, and Globalization in Samoa." 2006, February. Paper presented to Association for Social Anthropology in Oceania (ASAO) meeting, San Diego, CA.

Bourgois, P. (1996). *In Search of Respect: Selling Crack in el Barrio.* Cambridge, MA: Cambridge University Press

Brown, P.J., and M. Konner 1987. "An Anthropological Perspective on Obesity." *Annals of the New York Academy of Sciences* 499 (1): 29–46.

Brown, J.J. 2009. "When Our Water Returns: Gila River Indian Community and Diabetes." Case accessed September 2011 from the Enduring Legacies Native Cases website at www.evergreen.edu/tribal/cases. Specifically, the Pima case is found at http://nativecases.evergreen.edu/collection/cases/when-our-water-returns.html.

Browne, A., K.J. Strom, K. Barrick, K.R. Williams, and R.N. Parker. 2010, December. *Anticipating the Future Based on Analysis of the Past: Intercity Variation in Youth Homicide 1984–2006.* Report for the National Institute of Justice. Washington, DC: NIJ.

Butts, J.A., and H.N. Snyder. (2006). *Too Soon to Tell: Deciphering Recent Trends in Youth Violence.* Issue brief No. 110. Chicago: Chapin Hall Center for Children, University of Chicago.

Centers for Disease Control and Prevention. 2010. *Youth Violence: Facts at a Glance.* National Center for Injury Prevention and Control, Centers for Disease Control and Prevention. www.cdc.gov/violenceprevention.

Centers for Disease Control and Prevention. 2011. *Overweight and Obesity.* www.cdc.gov/obesity/data/trends.html

Davis, J. J. Busch, Z. Hammatt, R. Novotny, R. Harrigan, A. Grandinetti, and D. Easa. 2004. "The Relationship between Ethnicity and Obesity in Asian and Pacific Islander Populations: A Literature Review." *Ethnicity & Disease* 14: 111–118.

Douglas, M., and A.B. Wildavsky. (1982). *Risk and Culture: An Essay on the Selection of Technical and Environmental Dangers.* Berkeley: University of California Press.

Eaton, S.B., M. Shostak, and M. Konner. 1988. "Stone Agers in the Fast Lane: Chronic Degenerative Diseases in Evolutionary Perspective." *American Journal of Medicine* 84: 739–749.

Edberg, M. and Bourgois, P. Forthcoming. "Street Markets, Adolescent Identity, and Violence: A Generative Dynamic." In R. Rosenfeld and M. Edberg (Eds), *Youth Violence and Economic Opportunity.* New York: New York University Press.

Edberg, M. (2004a). *El Narcotraficante: Narcocorridos and the Construction of a Cultural Persona on the U.S.–Mexico Border.* Austin: University of Texas Press.

Edberg, M. (2004b). The Narcotrafficker in Representation and Practice: A Cultural Persona from the Mexican Border. *Ethos* 32 (2): 257–277.

Food and Agriculture Organization. 2002 January. "The Developing World's New Burden: Obesity," www.fao.org/FOCUS/E/obesity/obes1.htm.

French, S.A., M. Story, and R.W. Jeffery. 2001. Environmental Influences on Eating and Physical Activity. *Annual Review of Public Health* 22: 309–335.

Gardner, G., and B. Halweil. 2000. *Overfed and Underfed: The Global Epidemic of Malnutrition.* Worldwatch paper 150. Washington, DC: Worldwatch Institute.

Green, E.C., A. Jurg, and A. Dgedge. 1993. "Sexually Transmitted Diseases, AIDS, and Traditional Healers in Mozambique." *Medical Anthropology* 15: 261–281.

Gyeke, K. 1987. *An Essay on African Philosophical Thought: The Akan Conceptual Scheme.* Cambridge: Cambridge University Press.

Jeffery, R.W., and J. Utter. 2003. "The Changing Environment and Population Obesity in the United States." *Obesity Research* 11 (Supplement): 12S–22S.

Kaiser Family Foundation. 2005. "Mexican Immigrants' Health Status Worsens after Living in the U.S., Study Finds." *Daily Health Policy Report.* San Francisco, CA: Kaiser Family Foundation.

Khan, L.K., J. Sobal, and R. Martorell. 1997. "Acculturation, Socioeconomic Status, and Obesity in Mexican Americans, Cuban Americans, and Puerto Ricans." *International Journal of Obesity* 21: 91–96.

Knowler, W.C., D.J. Pettitt, M.F. Saad, M.A. Charles, R.G. Nelson, B.V. Howard, C. Bogardus, and P.H. Bennett. 1991. "Obesity in the Pima Indians: Its Magnitude and Relationship with Diabetes." *American Journal of Clinical Nursing* 53: 1543S–1551S.

Krug, E.G., L.L. Dahlberg, J.A. Mercy, A.B. Zwi, and R. Lozano. (Eds). 2002. *World Report on Violence and Health.* Geneva: World Health Organization.

Markey, S. August 8, 2006. "Obesity Explosion May Weigh on China's Future." *National Geographic News.*

McGarvey, S.T. 1991. "Obesity in Samoans and a Perspective on Its Etiology in Polynesians." *American Journal of Clinical Nursing* 53: 1586S–1594S.

Morland, K., S. Wing, A. Diez Roux, and C. Poole. 2001. "Neighborhood Characteristics Associated with the Location of Food Stores and Food Service Places." *American Journal of Preventive Health* 22 (1): 23–29.

New Jersey Office of the Attorney General, Juvenile Justice Commission. (No Date). *Gang Awareness Guide: Recognizing the Signs.* Trenton, NJ: NJ JJC.

NIDDK. 2009, November. "The Pima Indians: Obesity and Diabetes." National Institute on Diabetes and Digestive and Kidney Diseases. http://diabetes.niddk.nih.gov/DM/pubs/pima/obesity/obesity.htm.

Park, R.E. 1925. *The City: Suggestions for the Study of Human Nature in the Urban Environment* (with R. D. McKenzie & E. Burgess) Chicago, IL: University of Chicago Press.

Pollock, N.J. 1992. *These Roots Remain: Food Habits in Islands of the Central and Eastern Pacific since Western Contact.* Honolulu: University of Hawaii Press.

Reid, J. 1986. "Land of Milk and Honey: The Changing Meaning of Food to an Australian Aboriginal Community. In *Shared Wealth and Symbol: Food, Culture and Society in Oceania and*

Southeast Asia, edited by L. Manderson, 49–66. New York: Cambridge University Press.

Renzaho, A.M. 2004. "Fat, Rich and Beautiful: Changing Socio-Cultural Paradigms Associated with Obesity Risk, Nutritional Status and Refugee Children from Sub-Saharan Africa." *Health and Place* 10 (1): 105–13.

Sampson, R.J., and W.J. Wilson. (1995). Race, crime and urban inequality. In *Crime and inequality*, edited by J.H.R. Peterson, 37–54. Stanford, CA: Stanford University Press.

Singh, G.K., and B.A. Miller. 2004. "Health, Life Expectancy, and Mortality Patterns among Immigrant Populations in the United States." *Canadian Journal of Public Health* 95 (3): I14–I21.

Sow, I. 1980. *Anthropological Structures of Madness in Black Africa.* New York: International Universities Press.

Sundquist, J., and M. Winkelby. 2000. "Country of Birth, Acculturation Status, and Abdominal Obesity in a National Sample of Mexican-American Women and Men." *International Journal of Epidemiology* 29: 470–477.

Thrasher, F.M. 1927. *The Gang: A Study of 1,313 Gangs in Chicago.* Chicago, IL: University of Chicago Press

U.S. Census Bureau. 2009. *State and County Quickfacts.* Retrieved September 2011 from: http://quickfacts.census.gov/qfd/states/54000.html

van Dyk, A.C. (2001). *HIV/AIDS Care & Counselling: A Multidisciplinary Approach.* Cape Town: Pearson Education.

Vigil, J.D. 2007. *The Projects: Gang and Non-Gang Families in East Los Angeles.* Austin: University of Texas Press.

Weinberg, Z. 2000. "No Place to Shop: Food Access Lacking in the Inner City." *Race, Poverty and the Environment* 7 (2): 22–24.

Weismantel, M.J. 1988. *Food, Gender, and Poverty in the Ecuadorian Andes.* Philadelphia: University of Pennsylvania Press.

Whyte, W.F. 1993 (1943). *Street Corner Society: The Social Structure of an Italian Slum (Fourth Edition).* Chicago: University of Chicago Press.

Wilkinson, D.L., C.C. Beaty, and R.M. Lurry. 2009. Youth Violence: Crime or Self-Help? Marginalized Urban Males' Perspectives on the Limited Efficacy of the Criminal Justice System to Stop Youth Violence. *The Annals of the American Academy of Political and Social Science*, 623, 25–38.

Wilkinson, D.L. 2004. *Guns, Violence and Identity among African American and Latino Youth.* New York: LFB Scholarly Publishing LLC.

Wilson, W.J. 1987. *The Truly Disadvantaged: The Inner City, the Underclass, and Public Policy.* Chicago: University of Chicago Press.

WHO. 2011, February. *Obesity and Overweight.* Fact sheet 311. Geneva, Switzerland: World Health Organization.

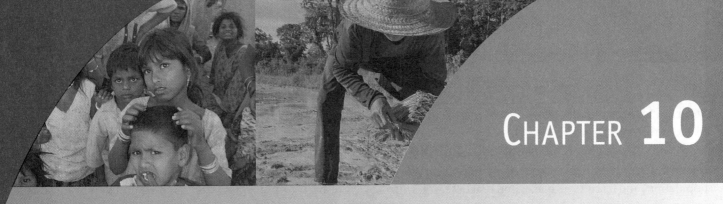

CHAPTER 10

A Primer on Research Strategies to Obtain Cultural Information

"There is nothing like looking, if you want to find something. You certainly usually find something, if you look, but it is not always quite the something you were after."

—J.R.R. Tolkien, from *The Lord of the Rings*

Suppose you are now out there working in a public health context. You could be working with a government agency or an international agency, trying to understand the prevalence of a health problem, or risk behavior related to a health problem. You could be a health provider trying to understand how to serve an increasingly diverse patient population, or you could be working with a private organization contracted to a funding agency to develop a health promotion program or communications campaign. Let's just assume that there is a cross-cultural aspect regarding the population(s) you are addressing. You have to find out more information about what's going on and why, and what role cultural issues may or may not play.

How will you do it?

One key strategy is developing partnerships with organizations that represent or work with the diverse cultural groups relevant to your work and can provide needed expertise. Another involves research—the collection and analysis of data—to help you understand these groups. In this chapter, we will focus on research.

Basically, there are two ways of collecting data you will need: 1) surveys and/or collection of other quantitative data (such as morbidity/mortality data from public health agencies); or 2) collecting qualitative data (from interviews, observation and other sources). Each has different strengths. Let's take a look at each of these strategies with respect to investigating cultural information of the type discussed in this book.

DATA AND PHILOSOPHY

To provide a foundation for understanding the two kinds of research, we are going to begin the discussion with a little philosophy. Talking about data and philosophy together is a very important starting point in being able to decide what kind of data you need and how to obtain it. As we now know, cultural data are very much connected to the marriage of meaning and practice—the way in which people's actions are almost inseparable from what they mean. This is information that is not often accessible, especially at first, by simply conducting a survey. Why? For one reason, to conduct a survey, you have to know what you are asking for in order to develop questions. Second, information about relationships between culture, meaning, and behavior are not easy to capture in yes-no or multiple-choice question formats. Perhaps most important, cultural information involves the way in which behavior is shaped and understood within systems of meaning. By nature, systems of meaning are subjective and interpretive.

This raises an important data question. In trying to establish facts or evidence about a population (or subpopulation) and its cultural beliefs and practices, you will have to come to some understanding about what counts as a fact. That's where philosophy comes in—because different kinds of data collection strategies (e.g., qualitative and quantitative) are linked to different (philosophical) ideas about what counts as a fact.

The conduct of research (which involves collecting data) and conclusions based on that research means producing an explanation of the events in question. Another way to think about this is that you are creating an *account* or *story* that explains the connection between certain factors and why the phenomenon in question (what you are trying to explain) is the way it is. That account will be judged as true or valid based on standards of evidence common within a research community.

Now we get to philosophy. Such standards are based on philosophical beliefs about facts, about how we know what we know—otherwise known as *epistemology*. In other words, the validity of explanatory accounts is based on an epistemology, which is a philosophical construct. In a Western, scientific paradigm, that underlying epistemology is closely connected to the philosophical schools of thought called *positivism* and *empiricism* that were central to the Enlightenment period in Western history and to the development of Western science. Here are two definitions (from MSN Encarta):

- *Positivism:* The theory that knowledge can be acquired only through direct observation and experimentation, and not through metaphysics or theology.
- *Empiricism:* The philosophical belief that all knowledge is derived from the experience of the senses.

In short, these epistemological positions hold that facts can only be determined through observation, experimentation, and that which can be experienced through the senses. To be a fact, something has to be tangible and measurable. That idea fits very well with the scientific method and generally with quantitative data collection

and analysis. But here is where we run into a problem. How can you see or measure subjective interpretation? How do you conduct an observable experiment? It's not easy to do.

So, back to philosophy for a moment. There were also other traditions during and after the Enlightenment period that differed from the positivists and empiricists. One of these is referred to as *phenomenology*. Here again is a definition (taken from MSN Encarta to be consistent):

- *Phenomenology:* (1) As a study of phenomena—in philosophy, the science or study of phenomena, things as they are perceived, as opposed to the study of being, the nature of things as they are; (2) As a philosophical investigation of experience—the philosophical investigation and description of conscious experience in all its varieties without reference to the question of whether what is experienced is objectively real.

The key to this epistemological school is the idea of things as they are perceived, and the setting aside of questions about objective reality. Now we are getting somewhere, from a philosophical perspective. If culture involves subjectivity and interpretation, it is very much about what people perceive. Remember our example of a classroom in Chapter 2? There were the objective facts—a rectangular room, with no windows, filled with people, and so on. Then there were the nonobjective perceptions about what those objective facts meant. For those who had a cultural idea, an available interpretation, that these objective facts meant *classroom*, they were instantly able to understand a lot about the situation, and to behave according to that interpretation. For the person who did not have a cultural idea (interpretation) of a classroom, he had to refer to whatever cultural idea he did have to interpret what the objective facts of four walls and the other "data" meant—and for him that turned out to be a prison room. That interpretation guided his actions.

You can see that in this example there is an interaction between objective facts and interpretive facts—the latter are facts about an interpretive process. These are different kinds of facts, yet important. When we are trying to understand the role of culture in health and

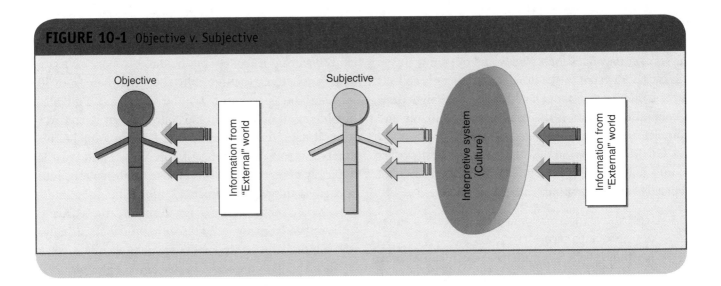

FIGURE 10-1 Objective v. Subjective

health behavior, the same principle that functioned in the classroom example applies. The objective or biological facts can be interpreted differently, and that will lead to different emotions, beliefs, motivations, and actions.

To understand interactions between culture and health, there are objective facts that are useful, but we need to understand the interpretive facts. Qualitative research methods are in part based on a phenomenological epistemology, on the idea that human beings are by nature interpreters, that much of what we understand as fact in the world is based on interpretation.

Figure 10-1 may help illustrate the difference.

DATA COLLECTION STRATEGIES

That's it with the philosophizing. Now we move to the nuts and bolts of data collecting. Going back to our two types of data, here is a set of definitions and descriptions to help illustrate the distinction:

Quantitative data refers to information that can be expressed numerically. This doesn't mean that the information itself has to be numbers, only that it is expressed that way. Quantitative data could include:

- Data from (quantitative) surveys, in which the responses to questions have a numerical value. For example, in a multiple choice question, each possible response is assigned a number; or if the

question is formulated as a scale, each point on the scale has a numerical value.
- Data that is in numerical form; clinical health data, for example, might include blood platelet counts or blood alcohol levels. Education data includes enrollment numbers by gender and test scores.
- Social indicator and demographic data, such as income levels, age, family size, and household members.

Quantitative data can be analyzed statistically in a descriptive sense (totals, like 94% of females in Country X are literate), or using a broad range of analytic procedures to establish correlations and other relationships among data items (variables). Quantitative data has the advantage over qualitative data in the degree to which it is generalizable. In other words, if you have a large set of health data or a survey that has collected data from a large number of individuals within a population, you very likely have reasonable evidence for making general statements about that population. At the same time, such data may be incomplete and not include key information, and those general statements could therefore be inaccurate. Institutional data such as health records can only support conclusions based on the information that is collected and stored. Survey data can only support conclusions based on the questions and response categories that were included in the survey. But what if there are other potential and meaningful responses to a particular set of survey questions? You would not know this in advance. Or what if the health data system only collects limited information about health risks? You might draw a conclusion based on the information available and completely miss an entire category of risk.

Qualitative data, on the other hand, generally refers to information that is not numerical in nature, and not typically expressed numerically.[1] This includes:

- Descriptive information about a process, a situation, an occurrence, etc.
- Attitudes, beliefs, opinions—which can also be investigated with quantitative methods (surveys), but only by setting up specific responses from which to choose.
- The nature and flow of social relationships.
- Emotions and cognitive understandings connected to real-time, daily occurrences, behaviors, and situations.
- Spatial data—the ways in which people's lives are geographically laid out (and conceptualized). This can be captured by quantitative methods as well, for example, with geographic information system mapping software.
- Subjective interpretations and meanings given to situations, events, people, relationships, and any other phenomena—in other words, understanding these phenomena from the perspective of the people/populations of interest.

Qualitative data are obtained from a different kind of research/data collection process than for quantitative data. The data are obtained from interviews, observations, participant observation, focus groups, ethnographic mapping, and visual recording of events, and from content and thematic or symbolic analysis of cultural materials such as stories, songs, tales, literature, or other media. These data collection methods are typically more inten-

sive and take more time than quantitative data collection. While developing a survey involves a lengthy process, administering it (collecting the data) is more or less a one-time activity that typically takes anywhere from 30 to 90 minutes per person. On the other hand, a qualitative interview may take several hours, or even extend over several days, for a single person. Prior to a qualitative interview, some time for building rapport and trust is typically necessary. The survey data can be entered into a database largely as numerical information; the interview data is most often text, not numbers, and is usually transcribed from an audio recording first before analysis. Importantly, while qualitative data usually involve a much smaller number of people and geographic area, there is an advantage of depth and breadth and more of a connection to the *natural setting* of the population or subpopulation than occurs with quantitative data—which is typically separated from its setting and decontextualized. Because of the smaller focus, it is harder to generalize the results to a large population. Finally, in a qualitative research effort, you are not limited to a predetermined set of questions, so the opportunity for collecting more complete and contextualized data is greater.

Qualitative and Quantitative Combined. Often referred to as a "mixed-methods" approach, it can be very effective to combine qualitative and quantitative approaches in order to use the strengths of each. The MidVille case in Box 10-1 is a good example. Without qualitative data to increase the contextual validity of the survey, the initial survey and its conclusions were not accurate, as noted. If a new survey was conducted in which the questions were grounded in the reality of MidVille's residents, the accuracy of its results would likely improve. In short, qualitative data collection is often important and even necessary in order to develop a quantitative instrument that is valid for the intended population. If you don't have appropriate response categories and questions on a survey, what can it tell you? Qualitative data can also be used as a parallel strategy, where a survey is used to obtain data that can be collected in fixed-response formats, and qualitative data is used for information that can't be captured that way—like the way in which a particular community coalition worked together or didn't.

---

[1] Though in some research methods where qualitative and quantitative data are both used, there are ways to convert or express information that is originally qualitative into variables that can be measured quantitatively.

BOX 10-1 Decontextualizing Data

Think of a hypothetical city named MidVille that has a highly transient workforce. People in MidVille are often from somewhere else, with attachments and backgrounds from their places of origin. Now suppose a polling organization comes in and conducts a survey about city issues, concerns, and local attachments. The survey finds a low level of knowledge about city affairs and a general lack of concern. Survey results are then compared to other cities and a banner headline reads: "MidVille ranks as most apathetic city in the United States!"

Is this information and conclusion true? Well, in a certain limited way it is. But it is decontextualized. It is information taken out of context and compared inappropriately to other cities where the residential and work patterns are different. The survey data are not connected to the reality of MidVille, and what they support is a misunderstanding about MidVille and its residents. In that sense, the conclusion is not true—or at least not accurate. To draw a more accurate conclusion, the polling group would have to take more time to learn something about MidVille—this might involve qualitative interviews with city government officials, with employers, and with residents. It might involve time spent at community events to get a better sense of local involvement patterns. With that kind of contextual information, pollsters could even go back and conduct another survey. This time, they wouldn't just ask about city issues, concerns, and attachments. They would also ask about length of residence, place of origin, and maybe something about the continued level of knowledge and concern MidVille residents had related to their places of origin.

The more contextualized banner headline might instead read, "MidVille's mobile workforce brings hometown concerns with them."

TWO EXAMPLES: CULTURAL DATA FROM QUALITATIVE INQUIRY

Imagine that there are two health-related research efforts designed to gather information useful in developing or improving programs. Ultimately, each one of these research efforts encounters cultural issues as follows:

Study One—A study investigating the connection between income and rates of diabetes in a specific state population, with a focus on diet.

Study Two—A study investigating the inconsistent utilization of healthcare services in a diverse metropolitan area, by demographic category and geographic residence of patient.

Study One. This study begins with the analysis of quantitative data on the state's population that was collected in a statewide health survey, looking for correlations between income level and diabetes. The analysis finds that there is indeed a correlation between low income and higher rates of diabetes, and it even provides a causal clue in demonstrating a correlation between low income and diet. This is all very important. But now we have to find out why these correlations exist. Here is where a qualitative research effort may be useful. The following is a brief summary of a qualitative effort that has that aim:

- Research team members visit a sample of primary care clinics in low income areas, and set up/conduct interviews or focus groups with a group of patients.
- In the interviews, researchers might ask what respondents typically eat for breakfast, lunch, dinner, or other meals. They could ask respondents to keep a daily journal, for say a month, about the foods they eat.
- Researchers might want to ask about awareness concerning the risk certain foods have for diabetes (e.g., high-sugar foods, high fat foods), and if that kind of risk is or isn't viewed as important.
- Researchers might even want to ask what people *feel* about the foods they eat. What does it mean to set out high-fat ham and potatoes for dinner? Maybe there are cultural traditions related to this meal, and maybe not. Maybe the respondents will reply with something like the following: "Well, we have a hard enough time providing things for the family [because of the poverty condition], so the least I can do is try to put out a good meal at dinner on the weekend, you know, something that really sticks to your bones."

What does this limited amount of information suggest? It may indicate at least one kind of meaning those foods have for those preparing and eating them in the context of poverty—as risky as they are for diabetes. The ham-and-potatoes dinner is *symbolic*. The respondents seemed to feel less than adequate in terms of what they could provide their families in general. A big "stick-to-your-ribs" meal was the only way they could think of to salvage that, at least a little, and allow them, for a moment, to feel like they were carrying out their parental role and being good providers. The operative concept here, gained from the qualitative research, is *being a good provider*. Food was directly tied to that role.

Even in this brief example, we can begin to understand the *why* that helps explain the correlation between diet and income revealed in the quantitative data. Can you use this information to guide a communications message about diet and diabetes (for this low-income population group)?

Study Two. Assume that an analysis of utilization data from the clinics (quantitative data) shows that people from certain neighborhoods close to the clinic did use the services, but usage from other neighborhoods just as close was low. Members of the study team are curious. Why would this be? A qualitative effort is launched to investigate:

- Team members decide that they will walk the neighborhoods before beginning a process of interviewing. During the walk, they loosely map out any characteristics of different neighborhoods that seem relevant to their research question. They notice that several of the neighborhoods appear to be primarily Caribbean in character—judging from the stores, signs, and people walking around. One of those Caribbean neighborhoods seems more established, in that it consists of solid row houses, a few Caribbean stores, and several churches—compared to the others, which have a higher density of stores and shops, hair braiding salons, restaurants (selling fish, oxtail soup, and roti), storefront churches, and a more active street life. They stop into a corner grocery store, and as one researcher buys a soda and snack, she asks the person at the counter, "If you don't mind my asking, where are most of the people in this neighborhood from?" Hopefully, this question prompts engagement in a dialog about several adjoining neighborhoods, which seem to correspond to different waves of immigration.

- Next, the contacts at the clinic have set the team up with two focus groups of neighborhood association representatives. In those groups, the neighborhood differentiation becomes a little more clear. The more established neighborhood is composed primarily of Caribbean immigrants from the earliest wave, who have been in the United States 20 years or more and whose children have largely grown up in the United States. According to community representatives, the clinic and its services are well known. There are two other neighborhoods whose residents tend to be recent Caribbean immigrants, and somewhat younger. The clinic is not well known there, and these residents often go to indigenous healers who can be accessed at shops and storefront churches. An additional set of interviews with shop and business owners confirms this, and reinforces the conclusion that these residents adhere to traditional medicine practices.

- Finally, a brief patient survey at the clinic also confirms that most patients are from the more established neighborhood. A researcher also asks clinic staff about traditional healers, and it is clear that no such healer has ever been at the clinic, nor have they been invited.

What does this information suggest? It looks as though the clinic is really only serving the neighborhood of long-time immigrants very familiar with and acculturated to biomedicine. That is why utilization (relative to the actual number of potential users) is low. What about the newer immigrants? There may be issues of insurance coverage involved, but the information gathered in the research suggests that the health practices newer immigrants are familiar with don't have much to do with the clinic.

One of the solutions we have talked about in previous chapters may prove useful here—increasing the collaboration between the clinic and indigenous healers. Doing so might positively affect utilization.

BASIC METHODS

Qualitative research strategies involve a kind of bottom-up approach, in which you begin with a relatively open-ended, preliminary inquiry and build knowledge through a succession of progressively more focused stages. Each stage is iterative—that is, it builds on the previous one, and knowledge can be said to *emerge*. By contrast, quantitative data collection tends to be more top-down in the sense that a survey doesn't so much build knowledge as confirm it or test its applicability to a population.

Figure 10-2 illustrates the qualitative research process, which takes the form of a pyramid.

Now let's take a look at a sample of basic qualitative methods. This is not a course in qualitative research, so the goal here is just to provide you an overall sense for some of the strategies that can be used.

Ethnography and Participant Observation

Ethnography and participant observation are classic qualitative approaches from anthropology. In their typical form, they can be time consuming and labor intensive because the goal is to spend time in the group or setting of interest in order to understand how behavior, beliefs, social structures, and cultural representations (e.g., sayings, symbols, rituals, art, media) fit together as they naturally occur. Ethnography and participant observation involve the following process:

- Establish a working, trusting relationship in order to collect in-depth data.
- Observe everyday activities (practices) and the relationships between activities.
- Observe activities in their natural setting.
- Observe the integration between activities, beliefs, and values.
- Observe social structures (e.g., families, leaders, healers, and faith organizations) and their relationship to activities and beliefs.
- During the process, collect a variety of in-depth data, including interviews, mapping, even quantitative data (e.g., daily counts of the number of people who are treated by specific healers in a community).

For public health and health promotion, ethnography and participant observation are usually employed in a much more limited context and with limited time frames. But the strategy can still be very useful in a number of situations and in combination with other strategies. For example:

- To understand the functioning of a community coalition: Attend all the meetings, observing and

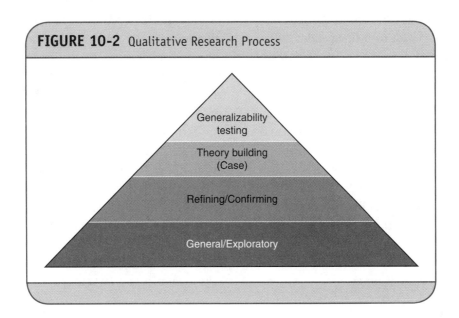

FIGURE 10-2 Qualitative Research Process

Generalizability
testing

Theory building
(Case)

Refining/Confirming

General/Exploratory

recording interactions, meeting accomplishments, barriers, and other occurrences.

- On a site visit as part of a health promotion project evaluation, to understand the activities conducted by the project: Attend/observe the activities, spending some time around program staff and clients, and try to get a sense of the interaction between the project and community.
- When cross-cultural healing practices are part of a particular context: Spend some time with indigenous healers, asking about and observing, where possible, healing practices.
- To understand the reception of a prevention practice or technology disseminated, for example, by community outreach workers: Accompany the outreach staff on their rounds in the community, observe and conduct interviews.

Interviews and Focus Groups

Interviewing is the "meat and potatoes" of most qualitative research. Conducting qualitative interviews is a different exercise than conducting a survey. Surveys involve a set question format, with a predetermined set of largely closed-ended response choices. In order to be generalizable and precise, they must be set up that way. Qualitative interviews have a different goal, and that is to generate information about something in a way that emphasizes respondent knowledge about it. In order to get that information, questions cannot have predetermined response categories; they have to be open ended, because an interviewer does not know in advance what respondents might say. The knowledge gained, in fact, comes from learning—over the course of many interviews—the range and content of responses. Here is another way to think about it: Respondents are cultural experts, and as the interviewer, you are a student. In that sense, when you conduct a qualitative interview, you are really trying to draw out the expertise of the respondent. There is a kind of relationship involved. Because of that, these interviews take more time than administering a survey, and as a result, the number of people interviewed (sample size) for a particular research effort is usually much smaller than it would be for a survey.

This is important for the study of culture and diversity in relation to health, because understanding people's subjectivity about health-related beliefs and practices is what you need to know. There are no right answers in qualitative interviews. There are simply respondent views.

In order to build your cultural knowledge about a population or group, there are several different kinds of interviews. Each type has a place in a sequence through which the information emerges, as in the pyramid in Figure 10-2. At the bottom of the pyramid, interviews are less structured and more fluid (because you have the least amount of knowledge at that point). The goal in that early stage is to begin the knowledge-building process. As you amass more knowledge and it begins to take shape, you can move to more and more structured and specific kinds of interview strategies, all the way up to formal survey interviews—using the latter when the purpose is to confirm or test what you have found in a larger population sample. The full sequence is as follows: informal/unstructured interviews, semistructured interviews and/or focus groups, and formal survey interviews.

Informal/Unstructured Interviews. These are best used when you really don't have much of an information base to work from—like the first informal discussions with shop owners in the clinic utilization study example earlier. In these interviews, you do of course have topic areas of interest, but you are not working with an interview guide or protocol. The interviews take more of a conversational tone, and may even be unscheduled. The answer format is open ended—focused on what respondents want to say about the issue. The purpose is to obtain leads and understand the basics—for purposes of follow-up.

Semistructured Interviews. Use this kind of interview when you already have a base of information to work from, either from previous informal interviews, previous work with the population or community, or insight from cultural experts. These interviews are more systematic and structured. Semistructured interviews are usually scheduled for a specific appointment time, and to conduct the interview you use an *interview guide* that lists the topics you want to cover, typically in the form of questions, but still with an open-ended response format. Before conducting semistructured interviews, it is important to identify a sample—that is, a description of the kinds of people you want to interview (e.g., community leaders, indigenous healers, community health workers, program staff, clients, or patients) and an estimate of the number of each type you think you will need to talk to. The sample description guides the recruitment of respondents. Like informal interviews, though, each interview may not be exactly the same, because—since responses are open ended—you are to some degree adjusting the question pattern based on what respondents say. You may even end up adding and changing questions as topics or information come out that you didn't expect. Though you can't be that flexible with survey interviewing, it is part of the learning process in qualitative research.

Focus Groups. Focus groups are a variation of a semistructured interview format that has both benefits and drawbacks. Focus groups are widely used in the development of communications/media campaigns (to develop and test messages and materials), in political campaigns, and in many public health contexts. Basically, a focus group is a semistructured interview done with a group, not an individual, and a group of similar individuals—people who represent a specific category of interest, such as adolescents from rural areas in Tennessee. The advantage is that focus groups provide a relatively "quick and dirty" snapshot of attitudes, beliefs, opinions, and in some cases behaviors of specific groups who are in the focus group sample. They should not be used when what you want are details of personal experience from respondents. They also can engender the *consensus effect*, which can be useful in some cases.

At the same time, focus groups require the management of group dynamics, which can be a disadvantage. Sometimes there are just a few people who speak up, and they may or may not represent the group. The focus group interviewer—usually called a "moderator"—has to control this and encourage more balanced participation.

Formal (Survey) Interviews. When you are finished collecting qualitative data and have reached a point where, even with open-ended interviewing, you are not picking up any new information, you may want to test

BOX 10-2 The Consensus Effect

Let's say you are conducting a focus group with people from a neighborhood about how often they exercise. [NOTE: Many times, to steer away from personal questions that could be awkward or improper in a group setting, focus group questions are phrased as "what do people like you typically do. . .?"] One person responds first, saying that people typically exercise 3 or 4 times a week. She might be saying this based on the *desirability effect*, the desire to give an answer that the respondent knows is the better or approved answer, though not necessarily accurate. In a focus group setting, other group members may chime in and correct this response, saying, for example "No, I think that's a little exaggerated. Most people don't exercise at all, or maybe just on the weekend. Only a few people I know ever do that regularly." If several respondents voice similar views, the original respondent may adjust her earlier answer, saying "Yes, maybe that is a bit exaggerated. But I do know a couple of people who do that, though."

Although this kind of consensus process has to be assessed carefully to be sure it's not just one or a few dominant respondents enforcing their view, it can provide a useful guide to accurate response ranges.

to see if the results of the qualitative investigation done intensively but with a relatively small sample are true for the group, community, or population as a whole. For this, it is often possible to convert the qualitative data into survey questions with a closed-ended format. In order to meet the goal of testing generalizability, survey interviews are conducted the exact same way each time, with a specific survey form and a statistically determined number of respondents (sample). Interviewers have to be trained carefully to minimize any influence on the respondent, or the survey can be administered via a laptop computer or the Internet.

Rapid Assessment Strategies

One combination research strategy that is used in both global and domestic contexts to gain a preliminary, but important, understanding of a particular health situation is called the "rapid assessment method." Typically, it is used when there is not enough time to do a longer study and when some relevant intervention needs to be implemented as soon as possible. The process is more or less as follows:

- Select knowledgeable intermediaries or stakeholders—conduct *key informant* interviews with them to gain a general lay of the land. These knowledgeable key informants are usually people identified by a local partner, local groups, or even the project funder, who are viewed as having significant knowledge of the health problem and population/group at risk.
- Based on what is learned from the key informant interviews, conduct interviews and/or focus groups with individuals who are members of the population of concern or individuals who have additional expert knowledge about them.
- In some cases, it may be useful to conduct brief, targeted observation to gain a better understanding of the community, community layout, or the context relevant to the health issue.
- Compare the findings from the aforementioned strategies to any other data that are available (e.g., from local health departments, clinics, tribal councils, or community organizations). Check to see if there are substantial discrepancies. If there are, go back and conducts another round of interviews/focus groups to identify the reason and reconcile the data.[1]
- Analyze the data and prepare a summary identifying the nature of the problem, key contributing factors for risk as well as protection (including culture-specific factors), with recommendations about a preliminary strategy.

Other Techniques

There are many other qualitative techniques used for identifying specific kinds of information. *Life history interviews*, for example, are semistructured personal interviews that seek an extended chronological history, allowing you to identify common patterns or trajectories. They could be used to learn about typical pathways to becoming an indigenous healer or shaman. *Free listing* and

sorting are techniques used to determine the items in a given cultural domain and how they relate to each other. This approach could be used, for example, to generate a list of culturally specific illnesses for a particular group and then to learn which illnesses are grouped together by cause and treatment—in other words the elements of an ethnomedical system. *Social network interviews* involve a very specific process for describing the composition of a group, the nature of relationships within the group, and the relation of one group to others.

For more information on these kinds of techniques, there are a number of good resources—see "Further Reading" at the end of this chapter.

RECORDING AND ANALYZING QUALITATIVE DATA

Data Types. Data from the kinds of qualitative research techniques comes in a variety of forms. Because interviews of various kinds are the most commonly used technique, the bulk of qualitative data will be in text form, as the notes or recorded transcriptions of interviews and focus groups. For this purpose, semistructured interviews and focus groups are usually audio recorded, using a digital recorder. Optimally, these recordings should be transcribed so that they can be entered into a text data file for analysis. Transcribing, however, is time consuming and/or expensive, so if resources are limited another strategy is to take notes and use the recordings as backup. There will also be times, particularly with informal interviews, where you do not have a recorder available, or the respondent does not want to be recorded. In that case there are few alternatives to good notes.

Other kinds of data include listings from free lists and tables or other depictions of the way free-list items were grouped by respondents, notes from observations (which can be formalized with observation guides or checklists), neighborhood/community mapping, and other formats.

Analysis. The goal of most qualitative analysis is to find common patterns and themes for a particular population or group. This could mean common patterns of health belief and treatment seeking, common views about health and risk, common understandings about the cause and meaning of a disease, common healing practices, common types of risk behaviors, and so on.

---

[1] This comparison process is known as "triangulation."

The use of the term *common* in this case refers to patterns that are shared to one degree or another (and part of the task is to document the degree to which such patterns *are* shared).

To get this from text, the most basic analytical process is *coding*. This is the task of marking, labeling and storing segments of interview text by what the segments are "talking about." In Study One earlier, as an example, interviews are conducted with clinic patients about their eating patterns, knowledge about diabetes risk, and then what (if anything) their diet meant to them—socially and culturally. The text from all these interviews would be stored and then retrieved for coding. The coding task involves:

- Going through the text and either marking segments of text by what they refer to (e.g., reasons for eating specific foods), or using a preset coding guide to find text that responds to the research questions.
- Creating files with all the text from all interviews (or all interviews within a specific category of respondent) that responds to each code.
- Analyzing the text within each code to identify response patterns, key themes, and most common reasons or practices for that group or for all respondents.

There are many software packages now widely used to conduct coding and analyze text. Two of the most well-known are:

- QSR NVIVO (from QSR International at www.qsrinternational.com)
- Atlas.ti (from Scientific Software Development GmBH, at www.atlasti.com)

There are also many other kinds of analysis. Free lists, for example, can be tabulated to identify most common items, the way in which respondents clustered or grouped items together, or most common rankings of items.

EXAMPLES

Here are just a few examples (from the author) about how these techniques have been used to identify cultural or other group-specific health beliefs, practices, and risk.

- For an HIV risk prevention study working with injection drug and crack cocaine users, interviews were conducted with a small sample of users (access was facilitated by health outreach workers) to identify social networks related to use, the nature of these networks, potentially high-risk intersections between drug use networks and sex partner networks, and how HIV risk related to injection and crack use was understood by respondents (Edberg et al. 1995).
- In one study to understand substance abuse and HIV/AIDS risk in three different Southeast Asian populations, qualitative research was used for three purposes: (1) Key informant interviews (with community organizations) were conducted in the first phase of the study to identify possible substance abuse and HIV/AIDS risk patterns in the three communities. (2) A series of focus groups were conducted in each community to identify (using free listing and sorting) the kinds of substances used and HIV risk behaviors, culturally appropriate terms for those substances or risk behaviors, and any kind of grouping of substance use by situation, gender/age, or other meaningful category, as well as groupings of HIV risk behaviors by similar categories. (3) This information informed the development of a survey which was then conducted in the three populations (see Edberg et al. 2002).
- In a project to develop an evaluation data system for a wide range of health promotion efforts funded by a federal agency that focused on health disparities of racial/ethnic minority populations, including immigrants/refugees, a two-stage qualitative effort was used. The stages included (1) interviews and focus groups with key informants who represented different types of grantee organizations funded by the agency; and (2) site visits to a sample of projects from each grant program funded by the agency—these site visits included interviews with project staff, observation of project activities and the community, and focus groups with project clients (see Edberg et al. 2003; 2011).
- In an ethnographic study on the U.S.–Mexico border to study popular media images of narcotraffickers and the connection between those images

and involvement in violence or other risk, participant observation and extended interviews were used to identify different media consumers and their respective interpretations of the narcotrafficker image, the meaning of that image to them, and any influence on behavior (see Edberg 2004a and b).

- In a study of risk for HIV/AIDS, sexually transmitted infections, substance abuse, and hepatitis among a sample of youth in Washington, DC, interviews, focus groups, neighborhood mapping (to determine youth knowledge about where local prevention services were), and a survey were used to identify beliefs about risk for these health issues, as well as behaviors, in different youth subgroups, among parents, and among community service providers (Edberg et al. 2009).

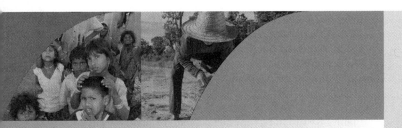

QUESTIONS

1. What are key differences between qualitative and quantitative research? What kind of data does each seek?

2. Why is qualitative research often most appropriate for identifying cultural information?

3. Name two key qualitative research techniques and their use in cultural inquiry?

4. Most quantitative data is expressed numerically; most qualitative data is in what form?

REFERENCES

Edberg, M. 2004a. *El Narcotraficante: Narcocorridos and the Construction of a Cultural Persona on the U.S.–Mexico Border.* Austin: University of Texas Press.

Edberg, M. 2004b, June. "The Narcotrafficker in Representation and Practice: A Cultural Persona from the Mexican Border." *Ethos (Journal of the Society for Psychological Anthropology)* 32 (2): 257–277.

Edberg, M., E. Collins, M. Harris, H. McLendon, and P. Santucci. 2009. "Patterns of HIV/AIDS, STI, Substance Abuse and Hepatitis Risk among Selected Samples of Latino and African-American Youth in Washington, DC." *Journal of Youth Studies* 12 (6): 685–709.

Edberg, M., K. Corey, and M. Cohen. 2011. "Using a Qualitative Approach to Develop an Evaluation Data Set for Community-Based Health Promotion Programs Addressing Racial/Ethnic Health Disparities." *Health Promotion Practice* June 15, doi: 10.1177/1524839910362035 (on line version).

Edberg, M., H. Klein, D. Clark, and J. Hoffman. 1995, June. "Variation in Size of Sex Partner Networks among Out-of-Treatment Drug Users: To What Extent Are IDUs a Bridge for Sexual Transmission of HIV?" Poster presentation. Joint NIDA/CDC Conference on Drug Use and AIDS, Scottsdale, AZ.

Edberg, M., F. Wong, R. Park, and K. Corey. 2002, July. "Preliminary Qualitative Results from an Ongoing Study of HIV Risk in Three Southeast Asian Communities." *Proceedings of the XIV International AIDS Conference*, Barcelona, Spain: World Health Organization, UNAIDS, Centers for Disease Control, and other sponsors.

Edberg, M., F. Wong, V. Woo, and T. Doong. 2003. "Elimination of Health Disparities in Racial/Ethnic Minority Communities: Developing Data Indicators to Assess the Progress of Community-Based Efforts." *Evaluation and Program Planning* 26: 11–19.

MSN Encarta. 2009. Microsoft. Retrieved from: dictionary.msn .com/.

FURTHER READING

Bernard, H.R. 2005. *Research Methods in Anthropology: Qualitative and Quantitative Approaches*, 4th ed. Lanham, MD: Altamira Press.

LeCompte, M.D., and J. Schensul (Eds). 1999. *The Ethnographer's Toolkit (7 volumes)*. Lanham, MD: Altamira Press.

Ulin, P.R., E.T. Robinson, and E.E. Toley. 2005. *Qualitative Methods in Public Health: A Field Guide for Applied Research*. Hoboken NJ: Jossey-Bass.

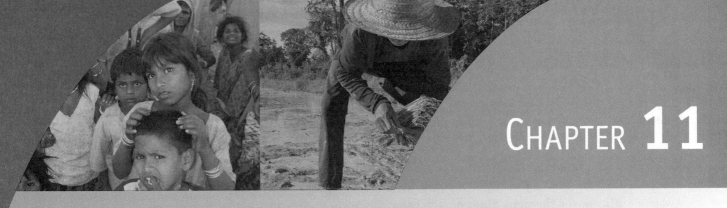

CHAPTER 11

Incorporating Cultural Knowledge in Health Promotion Interventions, with Selected Examples

"An ounce of application is worth a ton of abstraction."

—Booker T. Washington (1856–1915)

By this time, you have a sense of the role culture plays in human behavior, and a much more specific understanding of the ways in which culture impacts on health. Now we have to translate that into practice. What can you do with this information that will help improve the way health promotion efforts work across cultural contexts? One way to think of this is to look at what goes in to the *development*, *implementation* and *evaluation* of a program.

PROGRAM DEVELOPMENT

Unless the funder selects a program for you to implement (often the case in a global health context), this is usually the stage where you are either selecting a program that already exists (a model or evidence-based program), adapting an existing program to a particular population group, or developing a program of your own. How will you know which of these options makes sense? Unless you are partnered with a group or organization that already has expert knowledge of the population group you are working with, the likelihood is that you will need to conduct some *formative research*. Drawing on what has been covered in this book, for a cross-cultural effort, that formative research might need to provide answers for the following kinds of questions:

- Who are the populations/subpopulations involved?

- Are cultural factors relevant for the health problem of concern? Or are other factors (e.g., availability of insurance, transportation barriers) of primary importance?

- Does ethnomedical (or ethnopsychiatric) knowledge and practice play a role? If so, what are ethnomedical beliefs and practices related to the health problem being addressed?

- Who are the healers and indigenous experts related to the health problem? What do they say about it? How are they involved?

- Are there issues of morality or stigma connected to the health problem?

- Are there internal cultural factors (e.g., hierarchy, exclusion, marginalization, racism, gender roles) that create vulnerability?

- Are there any external cultural or political-economic factors (e.g., globalization, economic/social dependence, adaptation) that create vulnerability?

In Chapter 10, a set of research strategies was described (qualitative, mixed methods) that are useful in obtaining cultural information of this kind. These are, of course, very general questions about the role of culture. There will also be many other specific kinds of questions more closely related to the kind of program that is contemplated. For example:

- For a media or communications effort, it would be necessary to know what communications channels were significant for the population of concern, and cultural meanings associated with these different channels, as well as culturally appropriate constructs and language to use in communicating about a health issue.

- For a family planning intervention, it would be necessary to understand gender roles related to decisions about childbearing, gender roles in relation to children in general, gender-related concepts of fertility, how family planning decisions are made (in some cases, family members other than the couple may have a say), the composition of the household (multigenerational?), and to understand the kind of language best used to communicate about these often-sensitive subjects.

This kind of information is useful whether selecting an existing program, adapting a program, or developing a new one, and it may guide your decision about which of those options makes sense. If your formative research informs you that there are factors at work that no existing program addresses, then you are better off adapting or developing one if allowed by the funder. If your data fit right in with an existing program, that's very likely your best option.

Adapting or developing a program is a more extensive process. You have to take the knowledge gained in your formative work and translate that into program components, strategies, or messages. Then, in all probability, you will have to test out the new/adapted intervention a few times and make adjustments before anything begins to work as you planned.

PROGRAM IMPLEMENTATION

Program implementation is the nuts-and-bolts stage, in which the resources, logistics, plans, and people have to be mobilized to make a program function. It is the stage where assumptions that have been made about the role of cultural factors will meet their first test. You may encounter questions like the following:

- Are the individuals, groups, or organizations that were part of the collaborative effort actually collaborating as planned? Sometimes, there are factions, rivalries, or interpersonal issues that you did not expect. In one program working with several Southeast Asian refugee communities, for example, the author encountered rivalries that stemmed from generational differences in attitude about the home country government—reviled by the older adults who had escaped (following Communist takeovers in the mid-1970s), but less a preoccupation for younger generations.

- Are your conclusions about key cultural factors overstated or incorrect? Is this the result of your formative work, or is it based on information from the perspective of one person or group? Or is it simply because people and cultures are always adapting and changing? Maybe your original information about older adult preferences for traditional healers and younger generation preferences for biomedical practitioners turns out to be more nuanced, with some older adults in the community beginning to prefer the biomedical practitioners, and some younger community members wanting to return to their cultural roots.

- Are your understandings about the nature of a cultural community too generic or broad? Often there are many layers in a community that are based on class or other hierarchies, ethnic or regional differences, or immigration "wave." In one effort to conduct evaluation research on a program intended to increase access to care for Latino immigrants, the author and research team discovered that some of the discrimination and exclusion experienced by new immigrants from Central America came from Latino staff at the clinics, who were from other parts of Latin America, had been in the United States for a much longer time, and were much better educated.

- Do the cultural beliefs and practices of a marginalized subgroup you are working with present significant challenges in terms of the health problem being addressed? As we have discussed earlier in the book, conditions of marginalization and exclusion can have an impact on beliefs about risk and about priorities. These beliefs, practices, and priorities may not square with the public health goals of your program. What then? How will you maintain trust and try to find goals that make sense?

The basic message here is that when implementing a cross-cultural program, be aware and be flexible. Monitor the situation and maintain your relationships, because it is those relationships that help bridge gaps and solve problems that come up.

PROGRAM EVALUATION

Program evaluation can be enlightening, and it can be thorny. An evaluation involves the collection of data to determine if a program was effective, which, of course, can mean many things. Some evaluations just focus on operational or process-related goals and objectives. Did the program establish program XYZ as planned? Was a coalition created and did it hold together? Was a website created? Did a communications campaign reach the people it intended to reach? Others focus on longer term outcomes related to the health problem. Did the group or population change their HIV/AIDS risk behavior? Or their diet? Did more people access health care? Did the residents of a village use bed nets, and then was there a reduction in the incidence of malaria? Finally, some evaluations are intended to test a theory. If you claim, for example, that gender restrictions were a key obstacle for women in accessing mammograms, and your program sought to work with cultural leaders to find a tailored approach for increasing access, the evaluation may be a test of whether your diagnosis of the problem was correct in the first place. If you claim that a prevailing attitude of *fatalismo* (often seen in the literature) among a Latino population is hindering the willingness of people to make changes in diet, the evaluation may be a test of whether or not *fatalismo* is really as common as you thought. In any case, evaluations are an important part of the *cultural learning* that can take place when evaluating a health promotion program.

There are other key questions that come up as well when designing and conducting an evaluation in a cross-cultural setting. For example:

- What kinds of *measures* should you use to determine program effectiveness? Many existing questionnaires and scales are not appropriate outside of the Western context in which they were developed—in part because of the very issues discussed in this book concerning different understandings about health or different definitions of being well or not being well. Particular questionnaire formats may not make sense. Likert scales[1] are one example. Though common in Western survey instruments, many people outside of a Western setting are not accustomed to rating their experiences on a numerical or graded scale.
- Who determines the criteria for success? Is it a collaborative process with the population or community you are working with, or is it determined from the outside?
- What will you consider as data? Does it have to be numbers and figures? Does it have to be entered into a form? Can it be oral and narrative or visual? After all, there is a wide diversity in how people record and keep track of information, and some data formats just can't capture some of the subjective, experiential information that constitutes culture.
- How will you handle the social roles and potential barriers involved in conducting an evaluation—evaluators vs. the programs being evaluated—especially in a cross-cultural context, where evaluator/evaluated roles may intersect with mistrust and delicate social relations? How can the evaluation be treated as a collaborative effort?

FOUR PRINCIPLES FOR THINKING ABOUT THE INTERSECTION OF CULTURE AND HEALTH IN PRACTICE

Here are four basic principles to think about in applying the cultural knowledge discussed so far in this book to public health and health promotion interventions:

---

[1] Likert scales are survey questions that are often in the form of a statement, to which the respondent reacts by selecting a choice on the scale—for example, disagree, somewhat disagree, neutral, somewhat agree, agree.

- *Principle one:* Everyone, all peoples, have health knowledge and practices. These may or may not vary from the Western biomedical model. Either way, it represents a body of knowledge and practice that must be acknowledged.

- *Principle two:* The common situation is where more than one system of health knowledge and practice (ethnomedical) exists among a population or group. In other words, do not assume that where non-Western ethnomedical systems are prevalent, the biomedical system is not also known or acknowledged. Vice versa, do not assume that in Western culture the biomedical system is the only one people adhere to or believe.

- *Principle three:* The typical context of culture and health also includes a cultural ecology that has an impact on trajectories of illness/disease. This can include environmental, social, cultural, structural and political-economic factors that form a context.

The immediate significance of this context with respect to health behavior will vary.

- *Principle four:* If you consider the first three principles together, two important lessons are: (1) in order to maximize health outcomes in a given project, take time to learn something about the systems of health knowledge/practice that are part of the picture and work with them in the solution of the problem; and (2) take time to understand what cultural/ecological factors may impact on the health issue, and whether—or how—those factors can be addressed in an intervention.

CASE EXAMPLES

Now let's take a look at several global and domestic (United States) case studies of health promotion programs that were developed to incorporate cultural factors.

CASE 11-1

HIV/AIDS Prevention with Traditional Healers in South Africa

The Health Issue. As we have discussed in previous chapters, a number of nonbiomedical ethnomedical systems are common throughout Africa. These ethnomedical systems include personalistic elements (sorcery) as well as naturalistic elements and indigenous germ theory, and they incorporate a range of traditional healers. At the time of the project to be discussed, sub-Saharan Africa had already emerged as one of the hardest hit regions in the world with respect to HIV/AIDS.

The Project. In 1992, an HIV/AIDS prevention program was initiated in South Africa by the AIDS Control and Prevention (AIDSCAP) Project together with the AIDS Communication (AIDSCOM) project, both funded by the U.S. Agency for International Development. Drawing from the example of other pilot efforts at collaboration with traditional healers, the South Africa AIDS Control and Prevention Project trained an initial group of 28 traditional healers in both HIV/AIDS and sexually transmitted infection (STI) prevention. Each of these first-generation trainees would then train a second-generation cohort of traditional healers, and in turn each of those trainees would train a third-generation cohort.

Attendees at the workshop for the first set of healers represented five different traditional healer associations. This workshop included discussion of traditional healers' HIV/AIDS and STI beliefs and practices, general biomedical information about HIV and its transmission, prevention, potential indigenous risk and protective practices, HIV testing and confidentiality, education strategies, and other issues. These trainers-to-be were also assessed on their HIV/AIDS and STI knowledge, attitudes, and practices. Correct responses were adjusted to include indigenous terms in some cases—for example, it was correct to say that AIDS was caused by an *iciwane* (germ or virus) that "kills the body's soldiers" or *amasoja* (Green et al. 1995, 505).

The core trainer group then went on to train other healers. This second generation of trained healers was almost all composed of diviner mediums, known as *sangomas*, and was overwhelmingly female. The second cohort of healers then trained others. Interviews with a sample of healers revealed positive impacts of the trainings and workshops, a commitment to prevention, and generally positive experiences providing the education to their communities, even including condom demonstrations. There was some discussion in the interviews about traditional nonpenetrating, safe sex practices (for use, as an example, during menstruation) that could be incorporated in the prevention messages, but the general response seemed to be that young people did not know about or use these practices much anymore.

Results. This "snowball" process and its effect on each healer's patients as well as friends and family, was estimated to be significant. As of September 1993, 28 first-generation healers and 1,237 second-generation healers were trained, but only 245 third-generation healers were trained—for a total of 1,510 traditional healers. The team estimated that, if approximately 14 patients were seen per day, a total of 229,320 patients could have benefited from some prevention information regarding HIV/AIDS or STIs. One problem that came up during the project, however, was that the national traditional healer organizations turned out to be less than useful as collaborators because of jealousy and rivalries for power in the leadership. Instead, the local healer organizations, known as *impandes*, were more egalitarian and productive as collaborative partners.

Source: Green, Zokwe, and Dupree 1995.

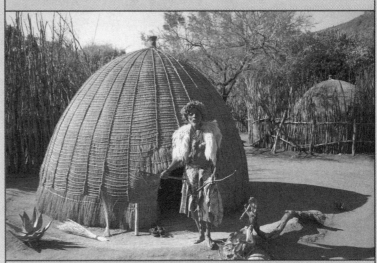

FIGURE 11-1 HIV/AIDS Prevention with Traditional Healers in South Africa

Source: © Attila Jandi/ShutterStock, Inc.

CASE 11-2

Improving Breast Cancer Control among Latinas

The Health Issue. At the time of the project described in this case, breast cancer was the most commonly diagnosed cancer among Latinas in the United States. Other research had also shown that Latinas differed in their knowledge about breast cancer more than other ethnic groups. In previous work, Chavez et al. (1995) had previously identified a Latina model of breast cancer risk factors that included trauma to the breast and "immoral behavior" (e.g., use of alcohol or drugs) as contributing to cancer—in contrast to the Anglo/Caucasian model that was primarily biomedical and genetic. Latinas were also more likely not to want to know or to tell their husbands if they had breast cancer, and had less general knowledge about risk factors, screening, and treatment. Therefore, Chavez et al. concluded that appropriate interventions addressing Latina cultural factors were needed.

The Project. The project team developed a cancer control program based on the idea of self-efficacy from Bandura's social cognitive theory (1986) and on the empowerment pedagogy of Paolo Freire (1970), viewed as appropriate frameworks within which to incorporate the Latina cultural models briefly outlined above. Together, these frameworks emphasize the development of skills and confidence, and participation in solving the problem of cancer prevention among Latinas, as opposed to a straight didactic teaching approach. In addition to the skills building (for breast self-examination, clinical breast examination, and getting mammograms), educational sessions were posed as questions to be answered by the group (about how to prevent breast cancer, what were the risks, etc.), and the group was tasked with coming up with solutions for breast cancer control.

Results. In an evaluation randomly assigning Latinas to the intervention or a control group, the women in the intervention group did increase their knowledge, their efficacy (confidence) about prevention, and their behavior in comparison to the control subjects, showing that the approach was effective. Program developers theorized that its success was a result of its cultural tailoring. The Latina women had relatively low literacy and were not highly acculturated to Western biomedicine or to formal didactic learning. The informal, group-based and interactive approach was able to engage them in the task of prevention.

FIGURE 11-2 Improving Breast Cancer Control Among Latinas

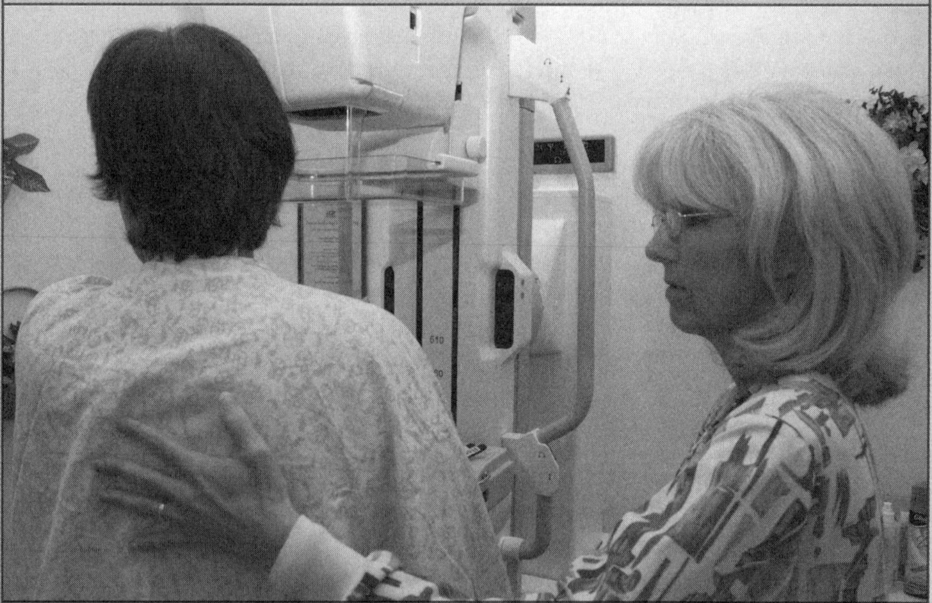

Source: Courtesy of Joseph Moon/U.S. Navy

Source: Mishra et al. 1998.

CASE 11-3

Addressing Cigarette Smoking among American Indians

The Health Issue. Though there are differences by region and tribe, American Indians have the highest smoking prevalence of any ethnic group in the United States at almost 41%. They also have a harder time quitting and so have lower quit ratios than other groups. Not surprisingly, cancer is the second leading cause of death for American Indians/Alaska Natives[1], and lung cancer is the leading cause of cancer deaths (Daley et al. 2010, 334). Smoking is also associated with other leading causes of death for American Indians/Alaska Natives, including heart disease and stroke (Legacy 2010).

The Project. A smoking intervention with American Indian peoples must first recognize that tobacco has long been a sacred plant, together with others. Tobacco has been used as a ritual symbol for peace and healing, for medicinal and religious purposes, and for instructional purposes. It is considered a sacred gift of the earth by many American Indians (Hodge 2001; Paper 1989). But traditional use of tobacco is not the same as cigarette smoking, either culturally or in the physical characteristics of use. It is used in controlled circumstances. Small puffs taken from a pipe, or participating in a cleansing ritual where tobacco is burned, for example, is not the same as the repeated, deep inhalation of smoke via cigarette use. For that reason, it makes cultural sense to think of the health problems as related to smoking or to chewing smokeless tobacco, *not* to tobacco in general.

The intervention has five components:

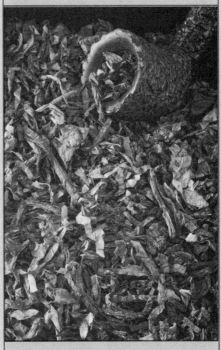

FIGURE 11-3 Traditional Sacred Tobacco—American Indians

Source: © iStockphoto/Thinkstock

1. *Qualitative, formative research:* Designed to involve participants in the development of the program—a community-based participatory research goal.
2. *Group sessions:* Group support for smoking cessation, led by a community member, not a counselor. The term *counselor* was not even used in order to reinforce the egalitarian nature of the groups and because that term implied a Western-trained individual and social distance between the group leader and participants.
3. *Telephone counseling:* There was some desire for individual counseling for issues not easily talked about in the group setting. The telephone counseling is still done by group facilitators, not licensed counselors. Motivational interviewing is used as a technique because it entails the involvement of the participant in identifying values and goals, followed by a self-examination of gaps between these values and participants' actual behavior—allowing participants to come to their own conclusions, not to be "informed."
4. *Educational materials:* These are designed with cultural issues in mind, not just paying lip service to American Indian culture by putting pictures of American Indian/Alaska Native people on what would otherwise be viewed as "white" materials.
5. *Pharmacotherapy:* When this was needed in order to quit, some participants were offered nicotine replacement therapy, varenicline (Chantix), and other products.

Results. According to their preliminary results, the self-report quit rate for the first 108 participants was 65% at program completion, compared to 25% at 6 months past baseline. Studies with other programs had shown much lower quit rates of 5–8%. The program developers note that the program was developed through a participatory effort that included both urban and rural American Indians/Alaska Natives, and that it was oriented to the cultural specifics of the participating peoples—the results might not be the same if used in a different context.

---

[1] American Indian/Alaska Native, or AI/AN, is the current title used by the U.S. Census and other agencies for this demographic category.

CASE 11-4

Adherence to Hypertension Treatment Regimens on the Caribbean Island of St. Lucia

The Health Issue. On the island of St. Lucia in the Caribbean, there is a very high prevalence of hypertension. St. Lucians were aware of the condition as a problem, and had for many years had a mixed medical system in which biomedical and traditional approaches coexisted for many years. The traditional personalistic system, similar to that in other Caribbean countries, is called "obeah." According to Dressler (1980), the sorcery that is part of obeah is not seen as sufficient to cause disease, though it may make it worse. Obeah practitioners are called "*jagajey*." If obeah is suspected as contributing to an illness, a healer called a "*gade*" is consulted to fight the obeah. The traditional St. Lucian ethnomedical system also includes naturalistic elements referred to as "bush medicine," which typically includes herbal tea remedies.

The Project. This was a research effort to determine the relationship between belief in obeah, bush medicine, or Western systems, and adherence to hypertension/blood pressure treatment. In formative research, Dressler and colleagues developed a survey to assess agreement/disagreement with traditional health belief statements, and then asked about the degree to which respondents had taken all or most of their last prescription in order to determine the relationship.

Results. Some of the findings were:

- The St. Lucian naturalistic system involves specific causes for specific conditions as they relate to a hot–cold balance and diet issues. They call hypertension "the pressure," and believe that it is caused by the chemical fertilizers used in the banana and other agro-industries.
- Dressler (1980) found correlations between naturalistic and Western systems, and between naturalistic and personalistic systems, but few similarities between personalistic and Western systems. So, the variance in adherence to treatment was correlated with belief in a personalistic system.
- Researchers also found that some individuals who had high English capability and level of education also expressed strong adherence to the personalistic system, contrary to expectations.
- Finally, the research suggested (corroborating other research) that adherence to blood pressure medication would be higher in St. Lucia if it were offered in liquid form, more like bush tea—which was used by individuals holding beliefs in both personalistic and naturalistic systems.

Source: Dressler 1980.

BOX 11-1 Family Planning in Albania—Interview with Laurie Krieger, PhD[a]

INTERVIEWER: Dr. Krieger, before we talk about a specific project, can you just summarize your background?

DR. KRIEGER: Sure. I am an anthropologist by training, and what you would call an applied anthropologist—that is, I use the tools of anthropology and the study of culture to help in addressing real-world problems, mostly in public health. My formal position title is Senior Advisor, Health and Social Science for an organization that develops, implements, and evaluates communications and behavior-related interventions in global health.

INTERVIEWER: So you work with cultural factors and health problems?

DR. KRIEGER: Yes. But I do want to say that in any situation I am working with, I don't consider the cultural factors to be barriers to health or something that necessarily needs to be changed. They are just an important part of the picture.

---

a. This interview is a composite from several discussions with Dr. Krieger about the project.

BOX 11-1 *(Continued)*

INTERVIEWER: Any examples you want to share of health projects where cultural factors were important?

DR. KRIEGER: There are many. But I'll talk about a USAID [U.S. Agency for International Development] -supported family planning project in Albania that involved the organization for whom I work, the Manoff Group, as well as the lead organization, John Snow, Inc.

INTERVIEWER: The floor is yours . . .

DR. KRIEGER: Well, let me start with a little background. In 2004, Albania had a low total fertility rate (2.1 lifetime births per woman), but also an extremely low rate of using modern contraceptives (8%). For family planning, most Albanians seemed to rely on withdrawal with abortion as a backup method. Relying on abortion tends to increase a country's maternal mortality ratio. So, there had been other projects trying to address this. They were more traditional information, education and communication projects, but they were only mildly successful.

INTERVIEWER: So you decided to try something a little different.

DR. KRIEGER: Pretty much. Because there was a limited amount of time for the project, we focused only on reaching married couples. Earlier research on this issue in Albania used surveys, individual in-depth interviews, and focus group discussions but didn't gain a sense of what the culture is or how to access it. For this project, we took a holistic view of family planning, situating it in gender identities, meanings, relationships within marriage and the family, notions of fertility, and practices and meanings related to sexuality—in other words, in its cultural context. Research on family planning in Albania was thin and no thick description[1] existed. Thinking of family planning as an expression and extension of relationships and meanings, and as needing to understand how it fit into Albanian cultures is different from the usual public health approaches. We assumed that family planning involves both thinking/emotion and practice, with a cultural aspect. To find out more about these, we used an ethnographic-style interview to get at cultural context and meaning of family planning and related subjects. The interview included a market research technique based on cognitive anthropology that asks the respondent to answer a question using pictures to represent how he or she thinks at an unconscious level, at the level of metaphors [see Zaltman 2003]. The research probed the meanings of various contraceptive methods to married men and women in our sample, and looked at gender roles and how they influenced thinking and action. The couples primarily relied on withdrawal, which to them expressed trust, love, and intimacy within marriage. Female respondents also mentioned that withdrawal limited pleasure. At the same time, these respondents, especially males, didn't know much about modern contraceptive methods, and what knowledge they had was often incorrect. For example, many perceived hormonal methods as harmful to women, likely due to the dissemination of limited, dated information about modern contraception by the former pronatalist (pro–high birth rate) government. Most respondents had discussed family planning and claimed that they made decisions on family planning jointly with their spouses. However, men's views usually dominated, despite the fact that women had more information about contraceptives than men.

INTERVIEWER: Did anything come of that research?

DR. KRIEGER: We used these results to design TV spots and programs, and an innovative pilot outreach program based on Outreach Negotiation Counseling or ONC. ONC was developed so that if successful, it could be scaled up to the entire country. Both research and program were designed with the premise that use of family planning in Albania is based on a continuum of decisions and behavior. The spots seem to have contributed nationally to moving people along the continuum to modern method use. Both outreach pilot areas showed an enormous increase in contraceptive acceptors: in one area, 56% of those visited at home by an ONC community nurse-midwife went to a service delivery point to at least discuss use of a modern method, and in the other area it was 65% of those visited.

INTERVIEWER: So trying to get at the cultural meaning of family planning helped design a more effective program.

DR. KRIEGER: Yes it did. But it's important to remember that the program had two other arms: training healthcare providers in family planning and also working with the Ministry of Health and others to ensure contraceptive security (a constant supply of sufficient contraceptive methods). Just communication alone could not have succeeded this well.

INTERVIEWER: Thank you so much for your time!

---

[1] "Thick description" is a term often used in reference to ethnographic and other qualitative description that includes significant information about cultural meaning as part of the description.

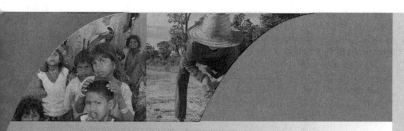

CHAPTER QUESTIONS

The questions for this chapter will be formatted a little differently than for previous chapters. Below are three different scenarios that need to be solved with culturally informed interventions. For each scenario, identify culturally relevant information, then propose a brief solution. The scenarios are fictitious.

Scenario One: Encouraging the Use of Oral Rehydration Therapy

The XYZ people on the island of XYZ believe that juvenile diarrhea is caused when a parent has forgotten to give the child a proper naming ceremony—that is, the ceremony at age 5 when the child is given his/her official family name. In that ceremony the naming is supposed to be accompanied by a basket of food presented as a gift to ancestors on both the mother's and father's side. However, one typical way to insult members of the father's or mother's lineage is to leave their names out of the ceremony. But if that lineage notices the insult, they might call upon a sorcerer to cause the child trouble, in the form of diarrhea. Curing is typically a combination of shamanic intervention and the use of medicinal herbal drinks. This has to be done with care, and by a trusted shaman, because the sorcerer may also try to slip the child a medicinal that will actually make the situation worse.

The easy cure for dehydration from diarrhea is the use of oral rehydration therapy (ORT), a packet of rehydrating substances meant to be mixed with water and given to the child. But XYZers have re-sisted the use of ORT because of their ethnomedical system and the possibility that the ORT is the work of a sorcerer. Yet XYZers do go to local medical clinics, for example, to obtain prenatal care services. The Western system, in other words, is also utilized for some conditions.

Question: What can you do to work with the indigenous system and yet provide the oral rehydration therapy to families? What would be your strategies/approaches?

Scenario Two: Smoking Intervention

Among the ABC peoples, smoking cigarettes is clearly a gender-based activity. Males smoke cigarettes from the time that they are 7 or 8 years old. Starting at that age is an unofficial rite of passage. Smoking is typically done at any occasion where men hang out, talk, and even work. It is rarely done by women, because it is viewed as a sign that the woman is loose and not well brought up. In addition, smoking and the type of tobacco used is usually talked about in the sense of a tradition, with certain tobaccos almost viewed in human terms, as challenges (e.g., "Okay, can you handle *this* one?").

General knowledge about cancer and other health problems resulting from smoking is known by many. But the knowledge of risk does not necessarily translate into preventive action (from a biomedical standpoint); in fact, it adds to the value of smoking, since smoking then becomes a known act of defying risk. This cultural view of smoking and risk is amplified by illness behavior common to men in which seeking help—especially prevention help when no symptoms are evident—would be viewed (by other men, anyway) as a sign of weakness.

There is a stop-smoking program in ABC territory, though. It is run by the brother of a high political leader, who got cancer from smoking.

Question: Your task is to increase utilization of the stop-smoking program via culturally tailored approaches. How might you do this?

Scenario Three: Improving Clinic Utilization

Middle City, USA, has become very diverse over the past decade or two. As a part of its effort to improve access to health care for residents of the state where Middle City is located, funds were allocated to build community health clinics in urban areas. Two were built in Middle City, and in the first few years, clinic no. 1 experienced a significant increase in use and seemed to be justifying its expenditure. Clinic no. 2, however, was not well used at all, and the state health department was puzzled as to the reason. Clinic no. 2 is located in a diverse and changing neighborhood that is composed of two population groups: (1) long-term residents who had largely emigrated from the Carib Islands (Caribbean area) 10 years ago or more, and (2) recent immigrants from the Seaward islands, very close to the Carib Islands and in many ways culturally similar. In general, the Carib Island immigrants came to the United States with resources, and were largely middle class and urban. The Seaward Island immigrants were more rural, less educated in Western-style systems, and came to the United States following economic difficulties resulting from a drop in the global commodity price of sugar, which was the mainstay of the island economy.

Your initial research has concluded that Seaward islanders did not generally have much access to Western-style health care in their home country. The indigenous health system included spiritual diviners, herbalists, and psychic surgeons, and health care was often provided in a communal setting.

Question: How might you increase utilization of clinic no. 2?

REFERENCES

Bandura, A. 1986. *Social Foundations of Thought and Action*. Englewood Cliffs, NJ: Prentice Hall.

Chavez, L.R., F.A. Hubbell, J.M. McMullin, R.G. Martinez, and S.I. Mishra. 1995. "Understanding Knowledge and Attitudes about Breast Cancer." *Archives of Family Medicine* 4: 145–152.

Daley, C.M., K.A. Greiner, N. Nazir, S.M. Daley, C.L. Solomon, S.L. Braiuca, T.E. Smith, and W.S. Choi. 2010. "All Nations Breath of Life: Using Community-Based Participatory Research to Address Health Disparities in Cigarette Smoking among American Indians." *Ethnicity & Disease* 20: 334–338.

Dressler, W.A. 1980. "Ethnomedical Beliefs and Patient Adherence to a Treatment Regimen: A St. Lucian Example." *Human Organization* 39: 88–91. [Also published as Dressler, W.A. 2010. "Ethnomedical Beliefs and Patient Adherence to a Treatment Regimen: A St. Lucian Example." In *Understanding and Applying Medical Anthropology*, 2nd ed., edited by P.J. Brown and R. Barrett, 263–268. Boston, MA: McGraw-Hill.]

Freire, P. 1970. *Pedagogy of the Oppressed*. New York: Seabury Press.

Green, E.C., B. Zokwe, and D. Dupree. 1995. "The Experience of an AIDS Prevention Program Focused on South African Traditional Healers." *Social Science and Medicine* 40 (4): 503–515.

Hodge, F.S. 2001, November. "American Indian and Alaska Native Teen Cigarette Smoking: A Review." In *Changing Adolescent Smoking Prevalence: Where It Is and Why*, edited by D.M. Burns, 255–262. Smoking and Tobacco Control Monograph 14. Bethesda, MD: National Cancer Institute.

American Legacy Foundation. 2010, October. *American Indians, Alaska Natives and Tobacco*. Washington, DC: Legacy for Health.

Mishra, S.I., L.R. Chavez, J.R. Magaña, P. Nava, V.R. Burciaga, F.A. Hubbell. 1998. "Improving Breast Cancer Control among Latinas: Evaluation of a Theory-Based Educational Program." *Health Education and Behavior* 25 (5): 653–670.

Paper, J. 1989. *Offering Smoke: The Sacred Pipe and Native American Religion*. Moscow, ID: University of Idaho Press.

Zaltman, G. 2003. *How Customers Think: Essential Insights into the Mind of the Markets*. Boston, MA: Harvard Business School Press.

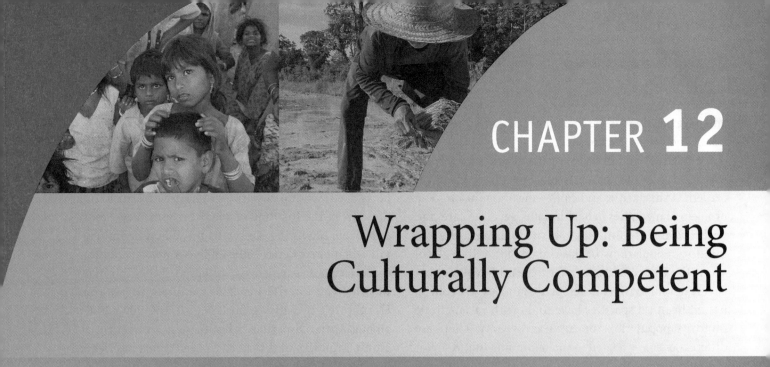

CHAPTER 12

Wrapping Up: Being Culturally Competent

"When your cart reaches the foot of the mountain, a path will appear."

—Chinese saying

What we have talked about in this book, in one sense, comes down to cultural competence. I say that with a caveat. The term *cultural competence* has been tossed around a lot in recent years, in ways that do not always do it justice. Being culturally competent has at times been equated simply with health information that is in the appropriate language, or that includes images or symbols said to be important for a particular cultural group. This can become very formulaic and one dimensional. It can also reinforce the idea of culture as something possessed by the *other*.

There is nothing inherently wrong with providing information in the right language and with cultural symbols. Language is important. Symbols are important. But what we have covered in this book should make it clear that negotiating and incorporating cultural factors in health promotion efforts is deeper than that, and more complex than that. Culture plays a role as part of the human social, symbolic, cognitive, and behavioral picture, just as biological factors do, or environmental factors do. In any given circumstance, with any group or society of people, you have to assess the way in which cultural factors are manifested, at multiple levels. Language and symbols may not be the only relevant cultural factors or the most important ones.

Yes, it takes a little more work to be culturally competent as described in this book. But it is well worth it, because any research conclusions you draw or programs you develop and implement are more likely to be valid and productive, even if more time or changes are necessary. And the human relationships formed in the process are of incalculable value.

In the United States, there have been major efforts in recent years to come up with guidelines and frameworks for cultural competence. Organizations like the National Center for Cultural Competence (http://nccc .georgetown.edu) and others have contributed extensively to the thinking about what this concept means and how it should be put in practice. The U.S. Office of Minority Health (OMH) and the Agency for Healthcare Research and Quality (AHRQ) contributed to developing the Culturally and Linguistically Appropriate Services (CLAS) standards as a way to help organizations shape their approach to cultural competence. These standards were published in the *Federal Register*[1] in December 2000

---

[1] The *Federal Register* is the official U.S. government daily publication for rules, proposed rules, and notices of federal agencies and organizations, as well as executive orders and other presidential documents.

and have become the basic reference point for organizational and program guidance.

The CLAS and other work in cultural competence was and is part of a larger national effort to address racial/ethnic disparities in health—meaning the ongoing problem of inequities in health status, access to care, and health-related circumstances between the majority and minority populations in the United States. In a global sense, the term could also refer to health inequities between developed/less developed countries. Of course, not all health disparities have to do with racial/ethnic minority populations or cultural diversity. There are differences solely related to socioeconomic status or, for example, geography (e.g., living in a rural setting with litle access to health care). However, the connection between diverse minority populations and health disparities is one key aspect of the problem.

Health disparities has been a central focus of public health efforts in recent years. Reducing or eliminating such disparities has been a major goal of both *Healthy People 2010* (U.S. DHHS 2000) and the recently released *Healthy People 2020* (U.S. DHHS 2010). The challenge of meeting this goal only becomes more important as the U.S. population grows more diverse and as the pace of global cultural interaction continues to increase. In the United States, health disparities became a central political and programmatic issue following the DHHS Secretary's Task Force Report in 1985 (U.S. DHHS 1985, called the "Heckler Report" after then-DHHS Secretary Margaret Heckler), and continuing through several reports documenting disparities in health care, including those from the Institute of Medicine (Smedley, Smith, & Nelson 2003); the Kaiser Family Foundation (e.g., Lillie-Blanton & Lewis 2005; Lillie-Blanton et al. 2002—the latter on disparities in cardiac care); the Commonwealth Fund (SteelFisher 2004); and recent National Healthcare Disparities Reports (e.g., AHRQ 2007; 2005), among others. Disparities in health status between racial/ethnic minority and majority populations have been documented over a wide range of health conditions (with variations depending upon the population and health condition—see, for example, www.omhrc.gov, the U.S. Office of Minority Health), and result from numerous and often interconnected causes (Edberg, Cleary, & Vyas 2010; Kawachi, Kennedy, & Wilkinson 1999; Starfield 2007; Williams, Neighbors, & Jackson 2003; Williams & Collins 2001). Thus disparities in health, as described, refer to disparities (differences in health status) that, as stated by Whitehead (1992, 433), "are not only unnecessary and avoidable but, in addition, are considered unfair and unjust."

CLAS STANDARDS AND THE KLEINMAN/BENSON APPROACH

The CLAS Standards. These standards (obtained from the U.S. Office of Minority Health, www.omhrc.gov), as noted, have become the key document used to guide cultural competence efforts in the United States. Let's take a quick look at the 14 standards included in the list. They are organized by theme: standards 1–3 address culturally competent care; 4–7 refer to language access services; and 8–14 refer to organizational supports for cultural competence. Another way to view it is that 1–7 are clinical or services-oriented, and 8–14 are organizational in nature (Fortier & Bishop 2003).

The first seven clinical/service oriented standards are:

Standard 1: Healthcare organizations should ensure that patients/consumers receive from all staff members effective, understandable, and respect-

---

BOX 12-1 One Definition of Cultural Competence

The following is one of the most widely used definitions:

"Cultural competence is a set of congruent behaviors, attitudes, and policies that come together in a system, agency or among professionals and enables that system, agency, or those professionals to work effectively in cross-cultural situations (Cross et al. 1989, 13)."

As you can see, this is highly oriented towards cultural competence as a *process*, as a set of things to do. Reference is made to attitudes, but the language of the definition is clearly pragmatic. There are other ways to think about this. We have gone into the issue in more depth, and in this chapter, a different definition and guidelines will be offered.

ful care that is provided in a manner compatible with their cultural health beliefs and practices and preferred language.

Standard 2: Healthcare organizations should implement strategies to recruit, retain, and promote at all levels of the organization a diverse staff and leadership that are representative of the demographic characteristics of the service area.

Standard 3: Healthcare organizations should ensure that staff at all levels and across all disciplines receive ongoing education and training in culturally and linguistically appropriate service delivery.

Standard 4: Healthcare organizations must offer and provide language assistance services, including bilingual staff and interpreter services, at no cost to each patient/consumer with limited English proficiency at all points of contact, in a timely manner during all hours of operation.

Standard 5: Healthcare organizations must provide to patients/consumers in their preferred language both verbal offers and written notices informing them of their right to receive language assistance services.

Standard 6: Healthcare organizations must assure the competence of language assistance provided to limited English proficient patients/consumers by interpreters and bilingual staff. Family and friends should not be used to provide interpretation services (except on request by the patient/consumer).

Standard 7: Healthcare organizations must make available easily understood patient-related materials and post signage in the languages of the commonly encountered groups and/or groups represented in the service area.

The organization-oriented standards are:

Standard 8: Healthcare organizations should develop, implement, and promote a written strategic plan that outlines clear goals, policies, operational plans, and management accountability/oversight mechanisms to provide culturally and linguistically appropriate services.

Standard 9: Healthcare organizations should conduct initial and ongoing organizational self-assessments of CLAS-related activities and are encouraged to integrate cultural and linguistic competence-related measures into their internal audits, performance improvement programs, patient satisfaction assessments, and outcomes-based evaluations.

Standard 10: Healthcare organizations should ensure that data on the individual patient's/consumer's race, ethnicity, and spoken and written language are collected in health records, integrated into the organization's management information systems, and periodically updated.

Standard 11: Healthcare organizations should maintain a current demographic, cultural, and epidemiological profile of the community as well as a needs assessment to accurately plan for and implement services that respond to the cultural and linguistic characteristics of the service area.

Standard 12: Healthcare organizations should develop participatory, collaborative partnerships with communities and utilize a variety of formal and informal mechanisms to facilitate community and patient/consumer involvement in designing and implementing CLAS-related activities.

Standard 13: Healthcare organizations should ensure that conflict and grievance resolution processes are culturally and linguistically sensitive and capable of identifying, preventing, and resolving cross-cultural conflicts or complaints by patients/consumers.

Standard 14: Healthcare organizations are encouraged to regularly make available to the public information about their progress and successful innovations in implementing the CLAS standards and to provide public notice in their communities about the availability of this information.

These standards have become a very useful tool in promoting the application of cultural diversity. At the same time, based on what we have covered in this book, the standards don't really address an improved understanding of the role of culture in health—and in fairness, they were not really intended for that. You won't learn about culture and health by reading or even abiding by these standards. But you will learn a range of actions to take to help ensure that cultural factors are addressed, and that is certainly important.

The Kleinman/Benson Person-Centered Approach to Cultural Competence. Arthur Kleinman, as noted in earlier chapters, is a central figure in the evolution of medical anthropology and cross-cultural practice. Peter Benson is an anthropologist at Washington University in Saint Louis who has worked with tobacco, globalism, and broad issues of cultural competence. Together, they offer a relatively simple framework for cultural competence that, like the CLAS standards, involves some process guidelines. But what Kleinman/Benson have included are processes that do touch on the kinds of relationships between culture and health we have discussed. Their framework is in part a reaction to formulaic approaches.

Cultural competence, they argue, should not be viewed as learning a list of "traits" that are supposed to represent a given culture. After all, individuals within cultures vary, and cultures are not static. Cultural competence should not be viewed as a technical skill or a checklist for clinician behavior. It is important in any situation to make an assessment of the role cultural factors play, because they might or might not be the central issue.

Their solution (Kleinman & Benson 2006) is a six-step process for incorporating cultural understanding in a health provider or program setting:

Step One: Instead of assuming, ask about ethnic identity and how much it matters to the patient. People "live" ethnic identity differently.

FIGURE 12-1 Doctor in Rural Clinic, Peru

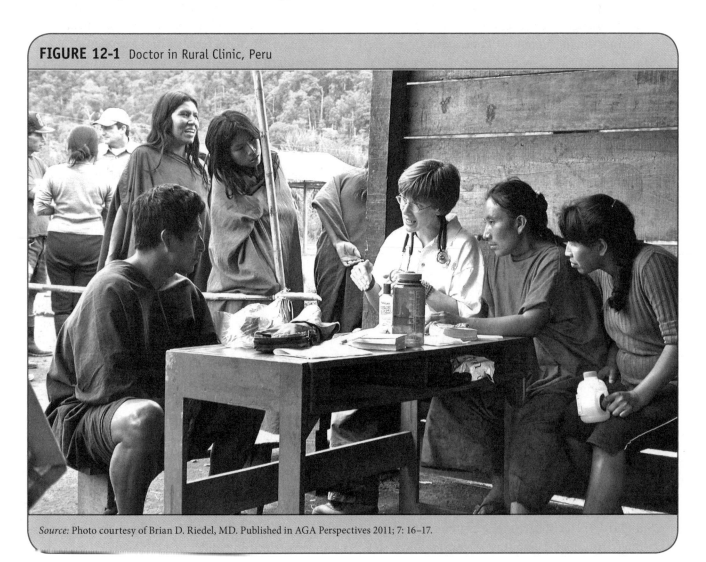

Source: Photo courtesy of Brian D. Riedel, MD. Published in AGA Perspectives 2011; 7: 16–17.

Step Two: Ask patients what is at stake for them and their close relationships because of the illness—this may include material, social, religious, or other consequences.

Step Three: Reconstruct the patient's *illness narrative*. What is his/her explanatory model about the illness and what it means? You can ask the following kinds of questions:

- What do you call the problem?
- What do you believe is the cause?
- What course do you expect it to take? How serious is it?
- What do you think this problem does inside your body?
- How does it affect your body and your mind?
- What do you most fear about this condition?
- What do you most fear about the treatment?

Step Four: Consider the ongoing stresses and social supports that characterize the patient's life. Suggest interventions/supports.

Step Five: Assess the influence of culture on the clinical relationship with the patient. Is it conditioning the way the patient responds or receives information/advice?

Step Six: Take into account the efficacy of cultural competency. Does it result in a good outcome? Does it obscure other contributing issues/side effects and produce a kind of cultural stigma?

You can see how this incorporates many of the themes we have covered—ethnomedical systems, sick roles, and the embedding of health problems in an ecology of social factors. The influence of this approach on how to think about cultural competence has had a significant impact at least in clinical settings, with medical journal articles taking up the theme (e.g., Carillo, Green, & Betancourt 1999), and websites such as Diversity Rx (www.diversityrx.org) serving as a portal for multiple resources.

A BROADER SET OF CULTURAL COMPETENCE GUIDELINES

Now let's try for a broader set of guidelines that refer not just to provider–patient relationships, organizational settings, or services, but to the entire scope of health promotion activities, from assessment to intervention and evaluation. These guidelines have to do with the basic interaction between culture and health and are based on the following definition of cultural competence:

> Cultural competence is an understanding of the role that culture plays in human behavior, health and otherwise, and the incorporation of that understanding in efforts to conceptualize health issues, conduct research on these issues, and collaborate to address them in practice.

We can frame the resulting guidelines as a set of principles:

Principle One: *Culture and health are bound together in the same way as are culture and other domains of human life—they are an integrated phenomenon.* As we have talked about throughout the book, culture is not an external object that somehow interacts with health or anything else. You have probably heard sayings like, "You can take the boy out of New York, but you can't take New York out of the boy." The culture–health relationship is like the second part of that saying—you can't take the culture out of health. Yet too often, the culture–health relationship is viewed as if culture is a discrete, external object that stands apart from a purely biomedical conception of health and can be put aside, blocked, or drawn into the picture as needed. Cultural competence under this principle means a basic acceptance of this integrated relationship as a given for *everyone*—provider and patient, public health bureaucrat and researcher, medical doctor and indigenous healer. It is neither good nor bad. It simply *is*. And if you accept this you are also more likely to treat people of all cultural backgrounds with respect, because everyone will be viewed, from a cultural perspective, as functional equivalents. You are also more likely, as a routine practice, to include assessment of cultural factors at multiple levels (as framed in this book), and their importance, or relative unimportance, in any given health-related effort.

Principle Two: *Culture is not an add-on, or a set of traits or items that can be pulled out of their cultural*

FIGURE 12-2 Principle One

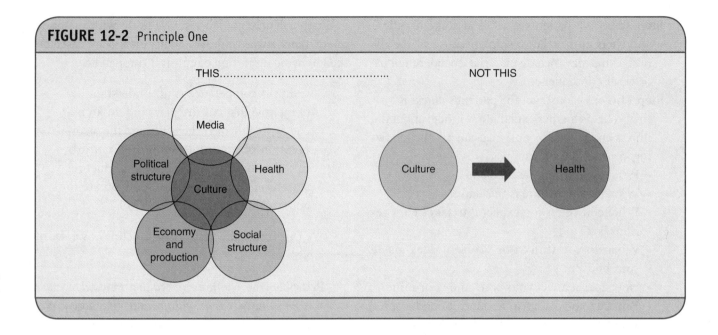

THIS... NOT THIS

context "just so." Take, for example, the construct of *fatalismo*, often said to be characteristic of Latino populations (Abraído-Lanza, Flórez & Aguirre 2007). This term appears a lot in the literature on cultural competence for Latinos. *Fatalismo*, in a health context, typically refers to beliefs among Latinos about a lack of control over events, related to a belief in divine will and determinism. But the research itself is not conclusive on the degree to which this is shared, nor on its impact on health behavior. Why? Because beliefs regarding *fatalismo* among Latinos cannot be separated from (in other words, they are embedded in) the degree to which Latino individuals are religiously inclined, have exposure to other ideas about causality, have power and resources, socioeconomic status, education, and other factors—the multiple levels at which culture operates. This doesn't mean it isn't useful to pay attention to the degree to which the construct is relevant for work with specific Latino populations, or to compare this construct to fatalistic/deterministic beliefs that exist in other populations, including Caucasian Americans. Cultural competence under this principle means that it is not helpful to treat cultural constructs as given, discrete items—in the same way you might say that "old Cadillacs have tail fins."

"Latinos have fatalismo" ≠ "Old Cadillacs have tail fins"

Principle Three: *Cultural beliefs and patterns represent something like central tendencies more than homogenous patterns.* Within a group of people or a society that shares the same culture, there will always be variation, based on other factors, including subgroup membership, socioeconomic status, marginalization, regional differences, interaction with other cultures, and responses to

FIGURE 12-3 1959 Cadillac with Tail Fins

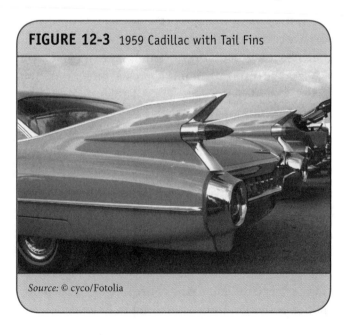

Source: © cyco/Fotolia

internal/external ecological constraints. What is important to realize is that central cultural tendencies act as a kind of shared text. Within the cultural group, people may disagree, dispute the meaning of aspects of the text, ignore others, or manipulate textual elements. But this is only possible if the text is generally familiar, even if knowledge of, or perspective on the details varies widely. Cultural competence under this principle means attention to both central cultural tendencies and the variations, and awareness of the basis for these variations.

A *corollary of principle three* relates to the participatory aspect of the CLAS standards. Yes, it is important to develop and provide services and programs as a collaborative process with appropriate cultural organizations and leaders. Principle three adds to that the caveat that it is also important to understand the cultural position of any particular organization of this type, because the cultural perspective represented by a given organization may be shaped by factors other than culture per se, including social class, region, nationality, occupational status, gender, recency of immigration and immigration experience, and others. Again, this is neither good nor bad. It just means that cultural competence requires an awareness of the general tendencies of particular cultures, as well as which version of a particular culture is "on the table."

Principle Four: *Cultures evolve as part of the world with which they interact—what may have been true about a given culture 50 years ago may not be so today.* The anthropologist Johannes Fabian (1983) authored a seminal critique about the way anthropology and other social sciences treat non-Western cultures, as if they remain fixed in time, as first described or imagined, instead of evolving and changing. He called this a "denial of coevalness" and argued that this practice reinforced the *otherness* of these cultures and peoples. Attempts at cultural competence have been guilty of the same distortion, where particular cultures are portrayed as static, or idealized, as something they once were. When the National Museum of the American Indian opened on the Washington, DC mall in 2004,

there was some controversy because the exhibits were not always historical or documentary in the way that exhibits might be in the Natural History museum. Instead, there were often exhibits of American Indians in contemporary life, who did not necessarily look like the "imagined Indian." The example is instructive. Cultures change, and being culturally competent under this principle means a regular effort to see and understand cultures as they are in contemporary settings.

Principle Five: *Cultural competence is practical, every day, and reality-based.* This last principle is an attempt to take the mystery out of cultural competence and of working across cultures in the context of health or any other domain. If you recognize culture as simply a part of the human makeup, it becomes culture with a small *c*. Normal. An everyday phenomenon. Yes, difference is involved, but difference does not equal exotic. Cultural competence often takes time and effort because it does involve learning, and it does involve collaboration and partnership, but no special gloves are involved, so to speak. Under this principle, cultural competence means being aware, but remaining human.

BOX 12-2 Cultural Competence—Five Principles

Principle One: Culture and health are bound together in the same way as are culture and other domains of human life—they are an integrated phenomenon.

Principle Two: Culture is not an add-on, or a set of traits or items that can be pulled out of their cultural context "just so."

Principle Three: Cultural beliefs and patterns represent central tendencies more than homogenous patterns.

Principle Four: Cultures evolve as part of the world with which they interact—what may have been true about a given culture 50 years ago may not be so today.

Principle Five: Cultural competence is practical, every day, and reality-based.

LAURA SMITH REDUX— COMPETENCY IN PRACTICE

When we left Laura in Chapter 1, she was in her room, on her bed, trying to make sense of the experience with an indigenous healer and a biomedical clinic in relation to the problem she was having. She was wondering whether or not to throw out the herbs and healing stick, especially now that she had a prescription from a doctor. *What was all that he said to me about seasons and balances and all that? But, well, it was kind of interesting. All the stuff about too much hot seasons—you know, in a way I kind of get what he meant by that.* She shook her head and decided not to complicate her thinking. *Never mind. I'm just going to lie down.* She fell asleep, and several hours went by.

Now let's return to the story.

It's late afternoon. All of a sudden, she feels very hungry, as if she hadn't eaten in days. *I suppose that's a good sign. But I guess I shouldn't overdo it.* Downstairs and a few storefronts away, there is a small restaurant and bar that looks decent and popular. Still feeling weak, she splashes a little water on her face, smoothes out her clothes, gives her hair a quick brush and trundles down the stairs from her room. The fresh air outside feels good, even if there is a little street dust in it.

At the restaurant, she sits down at one corner of the bar and asks for a menu.

She eyes the bartender. "Speak English?" Her words are not exactly distinct. The bartender nods. "Yes. What can I get for you? You . . . look like you could use something to wake you up," he says, smiling.

She pouts slightly. "A menu."

"Of course. You want in English?"

She nods. The bartender hands her a well-worn, laminated menu. Laura spots chicken soup and orders that right away—a familiar home remedy. And some bread, and hot tea.

As she waits for her meal, out of the corner of her right eye she sees a familiar face, with long gray hair tied in a ponytail. *Wait, who is that?* Her foggy recollection begins to crystallize, and she finally realizes that it is the healer she went to first. She keeps her gaze focused forward, hoping he doesn't recognize her. She has gone

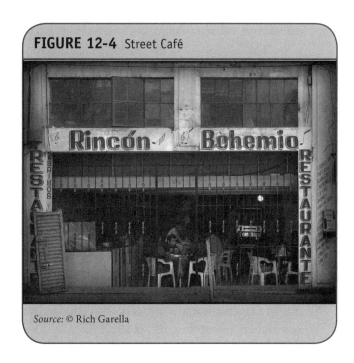

FIGURE 12-4 Street Café

Source: © Rich Garella

to a proper clinic and feels like she is done with that experience. *It will make a good story*, she thinks, *but once is enough.*

But soon, he taps her lightly on the shoulder. With a slight sense of dread, she looks up.

"Ah, the international manager . . ."

She is annoyed. "Well, yes, but that's not actually my name."

He shrugs and smiles sheepishly. "Yes. I know that. But I do not know your name. Would you care to tell it to me? I can see you are not so happy to see me, so of course you don't have to."

Laura calms down with his acknowledgment of her annoyance. "It's Laura. Laura Smith."

"Well how are you feeling, Laura Smith? My name, by the way, is Blas. Blas San Pedro," echoing her rhythm.

"Oh, not perfect, but a little better I guess. I went and got checked out and got a prescription for at least the nausea part." She wanted him to know that she had gone to a *real* clinic.

"Ah, you must have gone to the Fortuna Clinic around the corner."

"Yes. I didn't know that it was called that, but yes."

"Well, very good. I know them well. They do a good job. They even refer patients to me sometimes."

Laura is puzzled. She looks at him and squints, as if to underline her skepticism.

Blas laughs. "Ah, I see you are surprised."

"Well . . . I thought . . ."

"You think of me as a strange healer of native people, who would not be familiar with a clinic, nor them with me."

"Uh, yeah, well, I guess so."

"Can I tell you a little story? And please stop me if I bore you, or if you have a question."

The bartender brings her soup and bread. She turns and takes in a small spoonful. The warm liquid rolls down her throat and steam rises into her nostrils, opening her congested passages. *Oh, what the heck. I don't have anything else to do right now.* "Sure, go ahead."

"Very good. Many years ago, there were only healers like me in this town, and in most of the country. My father, and my aunt, and my father's mother, they were all healers like this. You could not just say you were a healer. Oh no. It took many years of working as an apprentice. No one would do that unless they had the gift, and the desire. Healers learned many things about what happens to people and why, and how three parts of the universe work together to make life do what it is going to do. But still, people got sick. People died from different diseases, sometimes when they were young. The healers were not perfect. Even my aunt, and one of my older sisters . . ." He looks off in the distance.

Sensing what he means, Laura interjects. "Oh, I'm sorry."

"Thank you. But that was long ago, though I still remember. Ah, where was I? Oh, yes, then maybe 20 years ago, some aid agency, I think first from a European country, then from the United States, came down here and set up a few medical clinics. At first, people were afraid to go there, but then they were happy, because the doctors seemed to fix some problems that the healers could not.

"And they had an exchange education program. I myself did this, against the wishes of my father. I went to a university out of the country for many years, and I studied psychology, and then began to study medicine, though I did not finish. I was excited at first, almost thinking that I myself was better than the healers in my own village.

"The good feeling about the medical clinics lasted just a year or so. Then there was a situation. One lady went to the clinic saying she had *bromo*, a problem we know about. I think the doctor did not have an idea about *bromo*, and he said she had a liver infection. He gave her a lot of medicines to take. She took them as he said, and she died. Some of the elders in the village went to the clinic and asked why she died, when she only had *bromo*. There was an argument. The medical doctor, as I heard later, got angry at the elders, and told them they did not know what she had. She died, he said, because she did not come soon enough. The elders said that the doctor gave her the wrong thing for *bromo*.

"Well, you see, this began a period where the feeling between the village and the clinics grew bad. People even broke the windows at the clinic. I was back from the university by this time, and was not sure what to do. I was confused. I knew about medical doctors, and I knew about healing. I tried one time to have a conversation with the people at the clinic. I have to say, in front of other healers from the village, they were insulting to me . . . and I don't think I was very kind in return.

"But after those disputes, I did not feel like anyone was right. They were not right. We were not right. And they did not know what we know. We did not know what they know. Why should there be a fight like this? There was one man, a medical doctor, who seemed more sympathetic than the others. One day, I asked him if we could have a cup of coffee and talk. He agreed. I told him that healers here have been treating people for more than a thousand years. We have names for the problems people have. We know what to do . . . and we know that we have limits. People here, mostly, are very poor. They have worked in the mines up there in the hills, or on farms, for a long, long time. They don't expect that every problem can be cured. But they understand what we do, and they know we are familiar with them and with their families.

"And I said to him, we do not have all the equipment you have. We do not have all the medicines. Our information does not come from scientific studies, but from experience—which, in a way, is like a scientific study. But you know that some of your medicines come from the same trees and plants that we use. And we have long experience with the spirit of the people, and what helps them, what is important for them. So why can't we help the people together? And that was all I said. The man sat for a long time and then said that he thought that was a very good idea. He said he was going to talk to some people. And he did. It took months, but we made an agreement with the medical doctors, and now we work together. Not all the time. But we, I, will refer people over to the clinics for some things. And they refer people to us for some things. So you see, it is not all as strange as you think."

Laura does not know what to say about all of this. It is far more than she expected to hear. "Mr. . . . Blas . . . why are you telling me all this?"

"Many reasons, I suppose. You know, I have a daughter, about your age. She is smart, too, like you. She went off to school. And she takes her healing stick with her, wherever she goes. It helps her focus when she needs it. And, maybe . . . you came to the healing center. I know it does not look like a doctor's office like you are accustomed to. I know you did not think much of the experience. But you went. Maybe you even listened. I give you credit."

Laura thinks to herself, *I did, didn't I.*

"Did you try the stick, the tea?"

Laura demurs on the question.

"I thought not. That is fine. You went to the clinic. But try it some time if you like. All those questions I asked you . . . they were to give me some knowledge about what else could be pressing you, helping the disease. I hope you feel better. And any time you pass through here, you are always welcome to stop by and to talk."

"Well thank you. I appreciate that." She is sincere, and taken in by his candor and gentle manner.

"Now I just want to ask . . ." Blas looks at Laura's face, awaiting a sign of permission to continue. She nods.

". . .International management. Of a business?"

"It could be. Of a business, or an international organization, or a nonprofit."

"Ah, so you will need these skills, to be able to understand many different kinds of people. It is very important now, to put yourself in other people's shoes. That is good."

"True."

"Well, then, I see that you are eating. A good sign. Good luck to you." And with that he puts on a cap and walks out of the restaurant, stopping at one or two tables to greet people before he leaves. Laura feels a pang, almost nostalgic, though of course this makes no sense. *Really, a very interesting man. People clearly know him, and in a good way, it seems. Not what I thought.* She scans the small interior of the restaurant as she finishes her soup and nibbles at the bread. Toward the rear, at one of those tables, there is a family, dressed like the native Indians she saw in the healer's office. At the other, a middle-aged couple in common Western-style clothing.

She heads back to her hotel, stopping briefly to pick up some gum from a vending stand. The street is a cornucopia, of sounds and people—dogs barking, cars honking, the buzz of small motorbikes. Vendors hawking wares or food to clusters of customers. People calling to each other across the street as if it were a small river running through the center of a village. Laura climbs the stairs to her room, and sits by the window, looking out at the scene again. The healing stick and bags of tea and powder are sitting on her bed.

Oh, why not. She grabs a bottle of water, pours it in a cup, and taps a little of the reddish-brown powder in the water, making a paste. As she was told, she rubs a little on her forehead and stomach. Very quickly she experiences an aromatic, cooling sensation, almost like menthol, that seems to work its way through her skin. With the window open, and the breeze flowing through, the sensation is very calming. Without thinking, she reaches over and picks up the healing stick, fixing her gaze for a few minutes on the obscure circular patterns inscribed in the disk.

Hmm. Maybe I was a little quick to judge. Really . . . I guess not everything is just like you expect.

The curtains flutter and she looks out the window again, at the early evening sun, reddish like the powder. She reaches over and puts the healing stick in her suitcase.

There was nothing else in particular she needed to do at that moment.

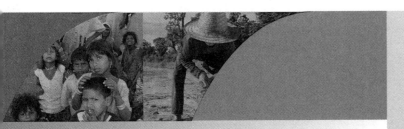

CHAPTER QUESTIONS

1. In this chapter, there are three sets of cultural competence guidelines. What are the differences among these three?

2. What is the connection between cultural competence and the issue of health disparities? Discuss this in both a U.S. and global context.

3. What do you think is meant by asserting that cultural competence is "everyday and reality-based"?

4. If you are designing a health promotion program, where does cultural competence as we have defined it fit in the process?

REFERENCES

Abraído-Lanza, A.F., K.R. Flórez, and A.N. Aguirre. 2007. "*Fatalismo* Reconsidered: A Cautionary Note for Health-Related Research and Practice with Latino Populations." Commentary. *Ethnicity and Disease* 17: 153–158.

Agency for Healthcare Research and Quality (AHRQ). 2005. *Third National Healthcare Disparities Report*. Rockville, MD: Agency for Healthcare Quality and Research, Department of Health and Human Services.

Agency for Healthcare Research and Quality (AHRQ). 2007. Program Brief: AHRQ Activities to Reduce Racial and Ethnic Disparities in Health Care. Rockville, MD: Agency for Healthcare Quality and Research, Department of Health and Human Services.

Carillo, J.E., A.R. Green, and J.R. Betancourt. 1999. "Cross–Cultural Primary Care: A Patient-Centered Approach." *Annals of Internal Medicine* 130: 829–834.

Cross, T.L., B.J. Barzon, K.W. Dennis KW, and M.R. Isaacs. 1989. *Towards a Culturally Competent System of Care: A Monograph on Effective Services for Minority Children Who Are Severely Emotionally Disturbed*. Washington, DC: CASSP Technical Assistance Center, Georgetown University Child Development Center.

Edberg, M., S. Cleary, and A. Vyas. 2010, February. "A Trajectory Model for Understanding and Assessing Health Disparities in Immigrant/Refugee Communities." *Journal of Immigrant and Minority Health*. DOI 10.1007/s10903-010-9337-5.

Fabian, J. 1983. *Time and the Other: How Anthropology Makes Its Object*. New York: Columbia University Press.

Fortier, J.P., and D. Bishop. 2003. *Setting the Agenda for Research on Cultural Competence in Health Care: Final Report*. Rockville, MD: U.S. Department of Health and Human Services, Office of Minority Health and Agency for Healthcare Research and Quality.

Kawachi, I., B.P. Kennedy, and R.G. Wilkinson. 1999. *Society and Population Health Reader, Volume I: Income Inequality and Health*. New York: The New Press.

Kleinman, A., and P. Benson. 2006. "Anthropology in the Clinic: The Problem of Cultural Competency and How to Fix it." *PLoS Medicine* 3 (10): e294.

Lillie-Blanton, M., and C.B. Lewis. 2005. *Issue Brief: Policy Challenges and Opportunities in Closing the Racial/Ethnic Divide in Health Care*. Menlo Park, CA: The Henry J. Kaiser Family Foundation.

Lillie-Blanton, M., E.O. Rushing, R. Ruiz, R. Mayberry, and L. Boone. 2002. *Racial/Ethnic Differences in Cardiac Care: The Weight of the Evidence*. Menlo Park, CA: The Henry J. Kaiser Family Foundation.

Smedley, B.D., A.Y. Stith, and A.R. Nelson (Eds.). 2003. *Unequal Treatment: Confronting Racial and Ethnic Disparities in Health Care*. Washington, DC: National Academy Press, Committee on Understanding and Eliminating Racial and Ethnic Disparities in Health Care.

Starfield, B. 2007. "Pathways of Influence on Equity in Health." *Social Science and Medicine* 64: 1355–1362.

SteelFisher, G.K. 2004. *Issue Brief—Addressing Unequal Treatment: Disparities in Health Care*. New York: The Commonwealth Fund.

U.S. Department of Health and Human Services (DHHS). 1985. *Report of the U.S. Department of Health and Human Services Secretary's Task Force on Black and Minority Health, Volume 1, Executive Summary*. Washington, DC: DHHS.

U.S. Department of Health and Human Services (DHHS). 2000. *Healthy People 2010*. Rockville MD: Department of Health and Human Services.

U.S. Department of Health and Human Services (DHHS). 2010. *Healthy People 2020*. Rockville MD: Department of Health and Human Services.

Whitehead, M. 1992. "The Concepts and Principles of Equity and Health." *International Journal of Health Services* 22, 429–445.

Williams, D.R., and C. Collins. 2001. "Racial Residential Segregation: A Fundamental Cause of Racial Disparities in Health." *Public Health Reports* 116 (5): 404–416.

Williams, D.R., H.W. Neighbors, and J.S. Jackson. 2003. Racial/ethnic discrimination and health: Findings from community studies. *American Journal of Public Health* 93 (2): 200–208.

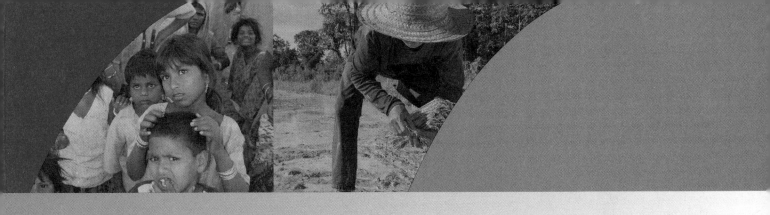

Index

Boxes, exhibits, figures, and tables are indicated with b, e, f, and t following the page number.